# YOU FORGOT
# TO MENTION

# YOU FORGOT TO MENTION

## TIPS for PARENTS by PARENTS

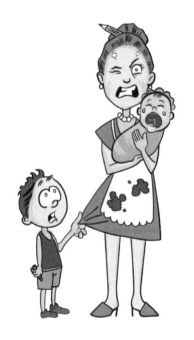

## Tiffany Parker

BROWN BOOKS
PUBLISHING GROUP

*You Forgot to Mention*
*Tips for Parents by Parents*

Brown Books Publishing Group
Dallas, TX / New York, NY
www.BrownBooks.com
(972) 381-0009

A New Era in Publishing®

Publisher's Cataloging-In-Publication Data

Names: Parker, Tiffany, 1989- author.
Title: You forgot to mention : tips for parents by parents / Tiffany Parker.
Description: Dallas, TX ; New York, NY : Brown Books Publishing Group, [2022]
Identifiers: ISBN 9781612545578 (hardcover)
Subjects: LCSH: Pregnancy--Popular works. | Prenatal care--Popular works. | Newborn infants--Care--Popular works. | Childbirth--Popular works. | Child rearing--Popular works.
Classification: LCC RG525 .P37 2022 | DDC 618.2--dc23

ISBN 978-1-61254-557-8
LCCN 2021921942

Printed in the United States
10 9 8 7 6 5 4 3 2 1

For more information or to contact the author, please go to www.BrownBooks.com.

*To all the beautiful moms and dads*
*who shared their experiences with me,*
*and to my amazing children*
*who gave me the personal experience*
*and memories I needed to write this book.*

# TABLE OF CONTENTS

# ACKNOWLEDGMENTS

I want to start by thanking my amazing husband for always encouraging me to follow my dreams, pushing me to believe in myself, and supporting my journey. I want to thank my kids, biological and bonus; if it wasn't for them, I wouldn't have the experience to write a parenting book. A HUGE thanks to my publisher, Milli—thank you for seeing my potential and being my corner man. Finally, to my editing team, y'all make a girl look good.

# INTRODUCTION

When I set out to write this book, I wanted to talk about all those things people don't mention (or only whisper about) when it comes to pregnancy. I first had this idea after I had my first baby, my son, Kenny. There were so many times I had no idea what to do for my baby, or something happened that I had never expected. When Kenny was just a few weeks old, he was constipated (or so I thought) and in so much pain. I had no idea what to do for him and felt terrible because I wasn't prepared to help my baby. I ended up buying a suppository to help him go. When my daughter was born and she became constipated, I did what I had done for my son and let my pediatrician know. He laughed out of sympathy and told me that it is extremely rare for exclusively breastfed babies to get constipated, as breast milk acts as a kind of laxative. Four babies later and I finally learned this. Where was this information when I was a young mother trying to help my baby (who actually wasn't constipated)? I kept wishing there was a book out there that could have prepared me for the unexpected, for everything that the other pregnancy books didn't talk about.

Then my second child, Andrew, arrived, and there I was again, experiencing new things for the first time and wishing again that there was a book out there that would provide me some answers. Never at any point in my life did anyone tell me that a parent and child could have bonding issues. So imagine my misery and horror when Andy and I didn't click immediately the way I had with Kenny. It took nearly six months for me to feel any real bond with my sweet baby. I felt guilty every day, and my feelings were a huge detractor in my already failing marriage. There was nobody that I could talk with about how I was feeling, and nobody to tell me that I wasn't the first person in history to deal with this issue. In that pre-social media era, I would have felt better just knowing I wasn't the only parent going through a bonding issue. Simply learning that you *do* eventually bond—or learning bonding tricks—would have had such a significant impact on me back then.

Four births and seven kids later (I gave birth to four babies total, and the other three are my bonus babies gained through a second marriage), I have learned that no matter how many kids you have, each time you are pregnant, give birth, and bring a new baby home, something will take place that will make you stop and think, *What just happened?* Just like in the rest of life, with babies there is always another surprise around the corner. I think God (or whomever you believe in) does this intentionally to keep us on our toes. One moment you think you are finally getting this parenting thing down . . . and the next you are lying in a puddle of baby vomit crying right alongside your new addition. Or you step out of the room for one moment, just to return and find that your toddler has used two hundred dollars' worth of makeup that you were supposed to be selling to paint his and his brother's faces (true story; you'll hear more later).

Not only am I a mom writing from the wealth of experience these seven kids have offered me, but I also have background in the medical field that has served me well time and again. I hope to offer some of that learning to you as well. Obviously, you should always consult your doctors and pediatricians with any serious and specific concerns, but I'm glad to be able to share some of what I've picked up in my years in the medical field. I'm a certified EMT as well as a certified nursing assistant. I started out in pre-med before choosing instead to focus on pre-hospital care. I've worked emergency rooms and in gynecology (so I've seen a lot), and I have a passion to share this side of my background alongside the personal parenting lessons I've learned or were shared with me by other parents.

Please remember, you are *not* the only one experiencing these trials, tribulations, and (most important) soon-to-be memories. I hope from this book you will learn that instead of crying when you see that mess of makeup everywhere, you think, "I need to get my camera." Because I assure you, that makeup won't matter in a year, but that picture will last a lifetime. Kenny, the son who covered his little brother in makeup, is fourteen now, and he still asks me to tell him that story again. We laugh about the things that, at the time, were the worst things I thought could happen. When someone posts on social media about their newborn being constipated, I help them out and relay a bit of information that took me far too long to learn.

Whether you are about to welcome your first baby or your fifth, this book provides firsthand tips, tricks, and funny stories to get you through pregnancy, childbirth, and the first few months with your new baby. The tips and tricks you read in this book are not things you will find in other parenting books. These are not your typical "and at twenty-seven days you want to . . ." recommendations. These are real stories from real parents who were right where you are at now and learned some valuable lessons worth passing along. Parents who have learned that sometimes the only thing that can get you through a tough situation is a little bit of laughter. So find a comfy spot to sit, grab some diapers (for the little ones, and maybe for you too), and hold on tight . . . this book will have you laughing, crying, and taking notes.

> It is nothing like what all the books say it is.
> —Michelle

# CHAPTER 1

# OUR BEST ADVICE

I cannot tell you the number of times as a new mom that I just needed to stop and catch my breath. Sometimes this meant taking a shower by myself or waiting until my husband got home and passing the baby off to him for a while so that I could (quite literally) do nothing. Other times it meant learning how to prioritize my responsibilities. Self-care sometimes meant the dishes didn't get done the second I felt they needed to, but that meant I was far more mentally prepared for my baby. Prioritizing my marriage while learning how to live life with a new baby meant that my husband picked up food on the way home so we could otherwise utilize the time it took to cook and clean up afterward. Sure, we didn't eat a home cooked meal, but I got a break, and my husband got a little extra time with his wife.

I remember calling my mom once, frantic, in tears, having reached my limit. My first son, Kenny, was crying and had been all day. I had not slept the night before and felt like I was going to lose my mind. At the time I was a seventeen-year-old stay-at-home mom whose husband worked from sunup until sundown. Partly due to my lack of maturity and partly due to my lack of sleep, I was at a point that I could not clearly define an appropriate solution. My mom, in her infinite wisdom, told me to put my son in the middle of my bed where he could not fall off, and go take a shower. She said the most beautiful words I had ever heard: "He won't die from crying."

I took my mom's advice. After securing my son in the middle of the bed, I took a shower. I spent that shower bawling my eyes out, regretting my decision to have a child. But I came out of that shower refreshed and found my little boy right where I had left him, peacefully asleep. I know that sometimes we as moms think we must put our needs behind the needs of our children. But at the end of the day, you cannot take care of your kids if you do not first take care of yourself.

I named this chapter "Our Best Advice" based on two things: first, my experiences as a mom; and second, how many parents recommended certain things (such as baby wearing). If more than a dozen people responded to my question with the same bit of advice, it made it into this chapter. That being said, you may see these tips sprinkled throughout other chapters, but they truly are the best advice someone can give a new parent. My own personal best advice is this: take care of yourself as much as you take care of others. No, I don't mean neglect your baby, but caring for your needs is as vital as caring for your baby's needs. This can be the difference between a good or bad parenting experience.

One simple example of self-care that you can practice in the midst of caring for a new baby is taking a deep breath when you start to become anxious or frustrated. Sounds stupid, right? Try it. We don't naturally use breathing as a relaxation method, but once your body gets used to self-regulating through breathing, it becomes easier and easier to handle those stressful moments. If breathing isn't your thing, try my earlier tip about taking a shower. I don't think people give the shower enough credit. Having that hot water pelting your back as your lungs take in the steam building up and having your mind overtaken by the sound of running water is the easiest way to relieve stress.

Typically, what people imagine when they hear the phrase "self-care" is that they are looking for a more "all-encompassing" self-care, such as going to a movie, doing their favorite activity (reading, painting, whatever), or going to do something just for them. This type of self-care may not be as plausible on a daily basis or even on a weekly basis, but it is still important to find time for these activities in your new life. Make a plan with your spouse, significant other, or someone close to you (if you are doing parenting solo) to take an hour or two to yourself. One thing I did as a single mom was trade these days with other single moms. I would watch their kids for an hour or two once or twice a month so that they could have some "me" time. In return, they would do the same for me. Now that I am married, I try to take some time for myself at least twice a month. After all, with seven kids, I could use a day (or twelve)!

Do not exhaust yourself with those house chores. They will still be there when you get to them. Your baby, on the other hand, will not be patient. Dishes and clothes can be done anytime. Take time for yourself when you can. Even fifteen minutes can feel like a vacation.

—Janine

# NEWBORN HEALTH AND PEDIATRICIANS

> Babies do not come with instructions! You are going to learn many things, especially with the first baby!
>
> —Rafael

I can't emphasize enough how important it is to ensure you have a pediatrician who truly listens to you and to your concerns. Even more important is having a pediatrician who has enough of a relationship with you to be honest and forthcoming. When it comes to caring for the health of your newborn, nothing can replace a frank conversation with a pediatrician you can trust.

About two months after my daughter was born, I rushed her to the doctor (again) for some symptom I was certain was fatal. She had probably coughed or something. Her doctor checked her out and gave her a clean bill of health (again). Next, he looked at me and asked how I was doing. I am not sure if he asked that because I was anxiously biting my nails, or because it was the second time in as many months that I had brought Layla in for basically nothing, or if it was because we had built up enough of a rapport that he felt comfortable asking. I told him how great things were, how lucky I was to have my little princess, and all the other things parents with newborns say. However, I finally gave up the charade and said, "Shoot straight with me, Doctor. Am I being an overly paranoid new parent? Be honest."

Even though Layla wasn't my first baby, it had been a long time since one of my boys was a newborn, and this was my first girl. In my head, I knew I was being extremely cautious and just a wee bit overzealous in my doctor's visits, but I needed someone else to tell me. Who knows? Maybe he would shock me and tell me that I was right in rushing Layla to the doctor every time she sneezed! The pediatrician smiled at me and said, "You are definitely being an overly paranoid new parent. But if rushing her to the doctor every time she coughs alleviates *your* stress, we are happy to see her. But you are doing a great job."

I am so grateful I had a pediatrician who was willing to be honest with me. Although he was never dismissive of my concerns, he was also willing to tell me when I was being a helicopter parent (as I apparently am when it comes to my daughter). If this doesn't sound like your pediatrician, find another one. Find someone whose opinion you respect, who also respects you, and doesn't care if keep him or her on speed dial. We all know the saying "it takes a village to raise a child," and I really believe that it is true. A good pediatrician is an indispensable member of that village. It's just as important to have people you trust when you need to ask for help as it is to remember to ask for help! Do not try to take care of everything by yourself. You will drive yourself and your baby crazy.

Trust your mom gut. You know what you are doing; you just do not realize it. When you are overwhelmed, take a deep breath, and do not be afraid to ask for help with the baby when you need it.

—Breanne

# THE LITTLE THINGS

> Do not use fingernail clippers on newborn nails. I ended up with ten bloody fingertips and spent the afternoon crying.
>
> **—Krystal**

I remember those days when I always had to make sure I had mittens for my little one. I was too afraid to cut his nails, but he would scratch his face up with his long nails if he didn't have mittens on. I was stressed about the scratches, and yet too worried to do anything that might hurt his tiny fingers. My mom came over one day and noticed how long his nails were. She had a solution that would never have occurred to me: she started biting off his little nails! At first I was shocked and disgusted . . . until I realized how well it worked. When she was done, his nails were short, I didn't have to worry about mittens, and most importantly, no blood or tears were involved!

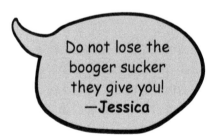

> Do not lose the booger sucker they give you!
> **—Jessica**

I know what you are thinking: *Ew, a booger sucker? What the heck is that?* It is actually called a *nasal aspirator* and it is meant to clear out your baby's nasal passage. A baby primarily breathes with their nose, so when their nose becomes clogged, it becomes difficult for them to breathe and eat. Imagine having a stuffy nose and your mouth taped shut so you are forced to breathe through your congested nose, and no way to resolve the issue. That is what it is like for a baby, but simply suctioning your baby's nose will help eliminate those problems. There are many different types of nasal aspirators on the market, including ones that require you to suck on a tube. I have not tried any of these (nor do I really wish to), but I never had to because I never had an issue with the aspirator we brought home from the hospital.

> On week three, my little one developed infant acne all over his face. I was horrified. But it cleared up after a few days.
>
> —Janice

Two to four weeks after birth, you may notice that your sweet little cherub is sprouting what can only be called "pimples." Either they are little red bumps or little white bumps, but it clearly looks like acne. Rest assured, these annoying little bumps are called *milia*, and are actually normal. Not only are they normal, but they go away on their own with zero medical treatment. As tempting as it is to pick at your little one's acne (well, it was for me), resist the urge. Although I don't know why they appear, I do know that popping or picking at those pimple-like bumps can cause scarring, infections, and even more bumps. Luckily, I learned this secondhand and not the hard way. My grandpa had large scars on his face that were caused when my great-grandmother popped those tempting little pimples. Understandably, they didn't know much about milia back then and couldn't just jump onto Google to look it up. The moral of the story here is this: best to leave these bumps alone, they go away on their own.

> Never hold your baby above your head after they eat. They can and *will* vomit all over you.
>
> —Lori

My mom gave me advice on this one too! It is her story that saved me from eating baby vomit. Yes, this is a thing, and most parents would say it is a rite of passage for all new parents.

Well, I am here to let you know that you can be a parent without this little experience! Babies spit up. You can't avoid it, but you can prepare for it. Playing with a baby directly after mealtime, tilting them, or not burping them after a meal will result in a partially digested milk shower. If you lie on the floor and lift a baby over your head right after they've eaten, know that they *will* take that opportunity to spit up and it *will* land directly in your mouth.

> When baby is teething or has a runny nose, roll a towel and place it under their crib mattress at the head of the bed. This helps fluids drain downward and not back into ears, helping prevent ear infection.
>
> —Meredith

My third son, Sylus, had terrible acid reflux and had to sleep in a tilted/inclined position. Rolling a towel and placing it under the crib mattress was a recommendation given to us by our pediatrician. An infant sleeping with his body tilted up (head above his feet) aides in fluid drainage and allows the fluid buildup from a virus or reflux to drain downward and not back up into their ears, where it could cause an ear infection. I will say this again, however—never do something solely based on a recommendation of a friend or a book. Always ask your pediatrician! This goes back to trusting and respecting your pediatrician. He or she can tell you what is right for your baby and warn you about any possible negative impacts. My daughter slept better in a tilted rocker, but these were recalled shortly after she grew out of hers because not everyone agrees with tilted/inclined sleeping.

# A LESSON IN COMPARISONS

Do not compare yourself to other parents.
—Leslie

Just understand that your first one is a guinea pig in a way. It takes time to learn how to parent, but by your second child, you feel like a pro.

—Dani

> Do not be in a rush for them to start talking, crawling, or walking. Once they start, they never stop. When you think you have figured it all out and have a great system or routine down, they switch everything up. The kid who loved PB&J one day will have a meltdown over it the next.
>
> —April

It wasn't until I had my fourth child, who was born ten years after my first, that I finally learned to let go of that nagging desire to compare my baby's development or my parenting skills to others'. Unfortunately, this isn't something that can be taught; it is something that is experienced and learned as you have children. I gave birth to my fourth child, a little girl, at the same time several of my friends were becoming first-time moms. Needless to say, my perspective by then was pretty different from theirs, and I wished I could make them slow down and enjoy every moment with their baby instead of pushing them to grow up faster. They were doing all the things first time moms do, but they should have been cherishing every stage of infancy because it goes by far too quickly.

We are all "this" mom, and if by some miracle you dodged this bullet, you know someone like this: With our first, we are confident that our baby was going to be the next Einstein, but by baby number four we just hope they don't hate us when they become adults. We feed our first child all organic, then by baby number four we are feeding them the french fry off the floor because it was on the ground for less than ten seconds. We try getting our first child to walk before the umbilical cord is even cut, then by baby number four we pray they don't walk before their first birthday. By baby number four, much like every other mom with more than one child (sometimes two), I discovered that all of those false pretenses were gone, and I wished I'd let go of them sooner.

Once you've let go of pretensions and over-the-top expectations, you're able to truly enjoy your time with your little one without wasting energy on comparisons. You no longer care whose baby does what first. Instead, you are just grateful that your little one isn't mobile yet because that means you get to hold them for that much longer. You don't care that they haven't started talking yet because that means he or she hasn't learned to talk back. Try to enjoy every moment with your new baby and don't worry about what is going on with other parents and their kids.

> Learn to say "No" and "No, thank you" and "Not right now" and "That's not really for me, but I'm glad it worked for you" and "Hmm, interesting" and "I don't think so."
>
> **—Annie**

> It is important to have someone advocate for you at the hospital.
> **—Katey**

> Cut yourself some slack. Do what you think is best for your baby and ignore the haters and, even worse, the well-intentioned critics.
>
> **—Susan**

There is a reason these quotes above are in this chapter, because they are absolutely the best advice outside of self-care. Heck, I would go as far as to say they *are* self-care. *You are allowed to say no* (although when you are a new parent, the world would have you believe differently). You are also allowed to have differing opinions. As a new parent, you will be guilted and bullied into doing things that you don't want to do or into doing things differently than you want to do them. You are allowed to advocate for yourself. If you can't, find someone who will. In the same way that we've all felt lost and in over our heads, every parent has moments when they feel that way too, and that is when someone needs to step in on your behalf.

When my daughter was born, I told the nurse that I didn't want the umbilical cord cut right away, I didn't want ilotycin (the clear stuff they put on newborns eyes) on Layla's eyes, and a few other things. These were not things that the nurse agreed with, and I hadn't previously told my ob-gyn. So instead of listening to my desires, in the chaos of the post-birth routine, the nurse did what she thought was best. There wasn't anyone with me that could stop her and advocate for me while I was too preoccupied to advocate for myself.

Just as much as you need someone to advocate for you, you need to be able to advocate for yourself and your family. You will meet the "world's greatest parents" along your parenting journey, whether they actually have kids or not, and they will be convinced they know the best thing for *your* baby. Oh, and they want you to know that everything you are doing, you are doing wrong. Ignore those people and trust yourself. Even if they are a "parenting expert," they don't know your baby. They have not been there with your baby twenty-four seven like you have. Trust yourself, and only seek advice from people that you know will give it to you straight.

When people give you unsolicited advice—which they will—you have every right to smile, nod, and tell them, "Thanks, but that isn't how we are going to do it," or whatever gets the point across. This is *your* baby, and you will do what you believe is right. Oftentimes for me, that meant that I would smile and nod, thank them for their wonderful advice, and go on my way . . . even if it was the worst advice I had ever received. If people thought they could do it better (which happened quite often with my colicky second baby), I'd pass him over and say, "By all means," knowing he'd be back in my arms in few minutes later and the well-intentioned critic would be on their way. I don't think people say or do things to be intentionally harmful or hurtful; they truly do think they are helping or being useful. But at the end of the day, a parent knows what is best for their baby . . . and if they don't, they will hopefully ask for help.

> You cannot spoil a baby by holding them. Do not listen to people that tell you, you are "holding your baby too much." That is NOT a thing. If your baby wants to be held, hold them. Show your baby that you will always be there to comfort them.
>
> —Molly

I cannot tell you the number of times in the last fourteen years that I have watched parents argue over whether they should keep holding the baby or put her down, let her cry it out or comfort her. This is what I have learned: you cannot spoil a baby. First off, when a baby cries, they are not trying to manipulate someone into holding them—they are trying to communicate. They might be tired, hungry, sad, hurting, uncomfortable, or maybe just plain lonely. Second, babies *need* love and attention. Love and attention lay a foundation for them to grow on emotionally, physically, and intellectually. It teaches them that there are people in the world that are reliable and can be trusted.

I'd like to tell you about my friend, Molly, who contributed of the above quotation. Molly is a woman who, despite never having had children of her own, advocates for holding babies and young children and showing them unconditional love and affection. She does this because she was not held as a baby; there was not somebody in her life that showed her consistent love in the form of touch. As an adult, Molly suffers from a medical condition called *attachment disorder*. Attachment disorder affects both children's and adults' ability to create or maintain healthy relationships with others, and is caused by inadequate emotional and physical connections with a parent or caregiver. Obviously, an attachment disorder goes beyond just not holding your baby all the time or practicing the "cry-it-out method," but it does teach us to appreciate how important physical and emotional connection is for a baby.

When a baby cries, they are experiencing stress in one form or another, and your child's stress level is something to pay attention to. Instead of associating crying with attention, start associating your babies crying with stress and think, *My baby is expressing to me that something is causing them stress, and as their parent, it is my job to figure out what that is.* As a mother of a toddler, I can tell you firsthand that what stresses my daughter out may not remotely affect me, but to her it is catastrophic. For example, every morning Layla wakes up and drinks "hot chocolate" (really, it's just chocolate milk) from a spill-proof sippy cup while she watches YouTube and mentally prepares for the day. I am not sure how this routine started, but for her it is a crucial part of her day.

Sometimes I forget to bring that sippy cup home from Doe-doe's (my mother-in-law), or we run out of milk, are in a hurry, or whatever else life throws at us in the midst of our morning routine. This disruption in Layla's morning routine is stressful for her, so she cries. For me, it isn't a big deal. She didn't get her hot chocolate, so what? I didn't get my coffee. But for her it is a really big deal. As her parent, I have to take that extra moment to recognize her stress for what it is and let her know that I support her. I show her I support her by simply giving her a little extra love or affection (usually in the form of extra cuddles or tickles) and offering up a solution, like letting her know that she can get some hot chocolate and go through her routine at Doe-doe's.

Although stress isn't always as simple as hot chocolate, when dealing with a newborn the solution is just as simple. They exhibit their stress by crying. As their parent, you are recognizing their stress by picking them up, giving them a little love, and trying to find the solution for their stress. In the next section, we are going to discuss stress and how catastrophic it can be to a parent, child, and even a developing fetus. It's too easy for us adults to go day after day with stress as part of the background, whether it's low-level or extreme, while never truly understanding how it is affecting our bodies both mentally and physically.

> The more stressed you are, the more stressed
> the baby is. Sometimes it is best to let someone
> else take care of the baby for a little bit, so you
> can have a break and relax.
>
> —April

Did you know the level of stress you feel during pregnancy negatively affects your unborn baby? I don't mean emotionally, I mean physically. A mother's stress can be fatal to a growing fetus. Crazy, right? Who would think that how you feel could be so detrimental to your unborn child? Well, when you are stressed, your production of certain hormones increases (cortisol and norepinephrine to be specific, for my medical friends) which affects your baby's development and can be fatal. Babies born to moms that experienced significant stress levels during pregnancy can be born prematurely, have lower birth weights, or even experience life-long effects. It is the mass production of these hormones that causes women to miscarry shortly after getting the news of their significant other's passing.

However, it isn't just unborn babies that can feel your stress. Your newborn baby can sense your stress, and it will stress them out too. The next thing you know, you will both be crying, overwhelmed, and questioning everything. We all have a threshold for how much we can handle. When you are running on very little sleep (as most, if not all, of us are when we have a new baby) that threshold is significantly lower. What we don't realize is how it affects our child as well as our ability to connect with and appropriately respond to that child. Know and respect your limits, and (I can't say it enough) don't be afraid to ask for help.

A nap or a shower may seem simple, but it may be all you need to feel refreshed and ready to face the day again.

As I close this chapter, I just want to say that none of us know what we are doing all the time. If someone says they have never felt this way, they are lying. We *all* have those moments when we feel like we are not good enough, when we have no idea what we're doing, when we experience a moment of sheer panic. My best advice to deal with these moments? Find yourself some mom friends who have been through all this (and are willing to admit it) and lean on their advice.

# CHAPTER 2

# MUST-HAVES

A must-haves chapter is so important in this book because new parents never really know what they need versus what just looks useful or cool. This chapter will hopefully save you a lot of time and headache when planning and preparing for baby while also helping you to create a baby shower gift registry. Let's face it: half the fun of being pregnant (and for some women, it's their only fun during pregnancy) is getting to have a baby shower and get all those fun gifts. But there's more to a baby shower than just cute outfits and the latest bottle dryer. You also want to be as prepared as possible before that new little one joins you. So let's dig in together.

## CLOTHES

One of the best things about being a mom (yes, specifically a mom) is changing your new baby one hundred times a day . . . their outfit, that is. Dads tend to just throw on clothes that cover all the right parts and go about their day, but for moms it's all about what looks the cutest, what will create the best photo ops, and what makes people stop and go "aww." That is, until it is 2:00 a.m., you are on night twenty-seven of no sleep, and you just mistook the bottle of lotion on the nightstand for your baby's bottle. Later there is a whole chapter dedicated to just how fun … and not fun … baby clothes can be. So of course, I had to add this topic to the registry list.

- Jammies (with a zipper—you'll see why later on)
- Sleep sacks
- Onesies with expandable neck openings
- Hand mittens for newborns
- Knit cap (if baby is born during cooler weather—remember babies lose their heat from their head)
- Socks

## MEDICATION

- Thermometer (okay, so it isn't really a medication, but still very necessary)
- Teething tablets
- Gripe water
- Baby Tylenol
- Syringe (usually comes in the box with the meds)
- Saline nose drops
  - I prefer Little Noses brand.
  - I recommend bringing home the bulb from the hospital and asking for a second one on your registry.
- Gas relief drops
  - I love Little Remedies brand.
- Baby Benadryl
- Glycerin suppositories (for constipation)
- Colic drops

# BABY CHANGING

- Diapers
  - o Buy various sizes! Nothing is worse than realizing in the middle of a change that baby needs to go up a size and you don't have them.
- Wipes
  - o Avoid scented wipes, as these could irritate baby's skin.
  - o I do not recommend wipe warmers, and here is why:
    1. Warm wipes will make your baby more likely to pee and . . .
    2. You cannot bring the warmer with you everywhere.
- Butt paste or desatin
  - o Pediatricians do not recommend baby powder anymore.

# BATH TIME

- Baby bathtub
- Baby washcloths
- Baby lotion
- Baby shampoo
- Baby towels

# FEEDING

- Dr. Brown's bottles
  - o Many people recommend Dr. Brown's bottles because they are advertised as being clinically proven to reduce colic, gas, and spitting up.
- Bottles that hold at least six ounces

- Slow flow nipples for newborns and fast flow nipples for older babies
  - Pro tip: I just used a safety pin to make my slow flow nipples become fast flow.
- Comotomo bottles
  - These are great bottles for babies transitioning from breast to bottle as it closely mimics the shape and feel of a breast.
- Medela bottles
  - These bottles hook right onto breast pumps for those moms that need to pump, then when you are done, you just unscrew the bottle off the pump and can put either a lid or a nipple on it.
- Nursing pads, either disposable or washable
- Nipple cream
- Burp cloths
  - You truly cannot have too many burp cloths.
- Formula dispenser
- Different shaped pacifiers


# BABY GEAR

- A Boppy pillow.
  - A Boppy is convenient from day one; it assists in propping up baby after eating to avoid acid reflux. It can be used to prop up baby when you are holding them, breastfeeding, or bottle-feeding. It assists in propping up baby after eating to avoid acid reflux. As your baby works to sit up, you can use the Boppy to protect your little wobbler.

If you are not familiar with a Boppy, it is a U-shaped pillow that tucks perfectly around your belly. It is great for nursing and bottle-feeding, but it is useful for so much more. Got a baby with a belly ache? Lay him on his belly with his head on the Boppy. Struggling with twins? Prop them up on the Boppy, and now you are free to feed both at the same time. Have an independent baby who is just not good at sitting up yet? You guessed it! Lean her against the Boppy. They even make a Boppy cover that has seat straps and helps baby to sit up more securely. I even used my Boppy to lay my babies on once they fell asleep so they could stay close to me, but I did not have to hold them.

> The Boppy pillow is my only "must-have" after three kids. It can literally be used for everything.
> —Amy

- Baby carrier (often called baby wear)
    - Twingaroo makes a double carrier specifically for twins

I wore my daughter in a baby sling pouch called a Hibiscusara front carry wrap that I could adjust to sit right across my belly. I personally have had many, many baby carriers, but I wish I had known about the Hibiscusara when my boys were infants because I never would have wasted my money on anything else. The carrier looked more like a purse than a wrap and was adjustable so my baby could lay high up to breastfeed or low down when I was walking (my movements allowed her to sway slightly and sleep). She would lay cocooned in there as if she were back in the womb, and slept for hours tucked into her little haven.

I flew, attended conferences and meetings, spectated my older kids' sporting events, and even took my boys to Six Flags. Throughout all these activities, nobody ever realized I had a baby in my "purse," not even when I flew from Dallas to Los Angeles. For me, concealing her in this sling meant not having to play "keep-off-the-baby" with all the well-intentioned people that always want to love on and touch new babies. The pouch also allowed me the freedom of having my hands free, while ensuring my daughter felt secure, nestled in the same position she had been in for the last nine months. She had spent nine months cocooned in a dark, secure space, being rocked by my every step. This pouch was the closest thing I could carry her in outside my womb, and it soothed her more than any of the other slings I owned.

> Any type of baby wearing [device]. Baby wearing is a life saver.
>
> —**Amy**

- Diaper bag
- A swing
  - I wish I had some magic ball that could tell you if your baby will swing from the side, front, or back. All babies prefer something different, but Fisher-Price has helped us out with that little dilemma. The Sweet Snugapuppy Dreams Cradle 'n Swing goes both directions.

# SLEEP

- Crib sheets
- Crib pads
- Receiving/swaddling/baby blankets
    - Although they have different names, they are all the same: small, thin(ish), cozy blankets perfect for swaddling.

Receiving blankets are another important go-to item for me. You may think you know how important they are, but you won't truly know until you've experienced how often newborns spit up. Any time I burped my baby, I'd toss a receiving blanket over my shoulder. This saved my clothes from getting spit-up on them a million times. Then I'd toss the dirty blanket in a bag and pull out a clean one. I never left home with less than a dozen receiving blankets, and they were strategically placed all over the house! Now that my daughter is a toddler, she uses her old receiving blankets for her dolls.

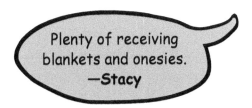

Plenty of receiving blankets and onesies. —Stacy

# SAFETY

- Head, neck, and body support pillow
    - This pillow is intended for the car seat and protects your baby's head from flopping around. I prefer the

ones that are three-in-one and grow with your baby. You will feel better with your new baby's head secure and supported.

- Nail clippers
  - o I prefer Safety 1st brand.

Although you won't need to babyproof your house until baby becomes mobile, it is always nice to ask for the things you will need so you have one less thing to worry about.

- Cabinet locks
- Sharp edge covers
- Doorknob covers
- Outlet plug protectors
- Toilet locks
- Baby monitor
- Furniture straps

Although you may not be asking for these next two items for your baby shower, they are still important for your overall comfort as a new parent.

My must-have would be snacks in main rooms. You never know when baby will fall asleep, and you will want food close at all times.

—April

I absolutely needed water by my side when I nursed. It was inevitable that the moment I started nursing, my mouth would get dry, and I would be wishing I had a glass of water.

—Whitney

Nursing takes a lot out of you, believe it or not. I remember at my six-week postpartum appointment with my son, Kenny, I was nursing in the waiting room while I waited for the doctor. About the time that I realized I was so thirsty I could spit dust, a nurse came out and offered me a glass of water. I guess the look on my face asked the question my mouth hadn't, because she smiled and told me how thirsty moms get when nursing. She wasn't kidding either: every time I nursed, I would get incredibly thirsty. So I started making sure I always had a water bottle nearby so I could hydrate as my little one sucked out all my hydration. Later, I learned that you get thirsty thanks to the production of oxytocin in your brain. It is your body's way of making you drink more water so that you can produce more breast milk.

Sitting down to nurse may be the only time(s) during the day that you get to take a bit of a break and just relax for a moment. Whether you are running around after other kids, taking care of the household, or just have your hands full with your new baby, you likely forget to take some time to reenergize yourself, specifically in the form of eating. There isn't much you can do while nursing besides check your phone, catch up on some TV, or take a thousand nursing pictures, so it is nice to take that time to eat a snack and reenergize yourself. Keeping snacks in your diaper bag or the rooms in which you typically breastfeed means you won't have to shuffle around trying to find something to eat while juggling a nursing baby.

You absolutely need a postpartum upside-down peri bottle. You will not want to wipe or even touch anywhere down there. If you get stitches, it stings when you pee. I would put warm water in this to help me go and to clean up afterward.
—Savannah

A girdle-like waist cinch will help with postpartum healing.
—Kristi

If you give birth vaginally, then there is a strong likelihood that you will tear your vagina or require an episiotomy (where they cut you between your vagina and anus to make the opening of your vagina bigger). If one of the two occurs, they will stitch you up in the minutes following your delivery, and for roughly the first six weeks you will not want to touch your vaginal area, let alone wipe it. The hospital helps with the pain by providing a peri bottle, lidocaine spray (numbing spray), and bags of ice, which you can bring home after you are released from the hospital. A peri bottle is essentially a water bottle you squeeze to shoot out water. After birth, you use it in lieu of toilet paper so that you don't irritate your stitches or recently stretched skin.

If you fill the bottle with warm water, it helps sooth the burning or itching while also cleaning the area. Spray some numbing spray on afterward, toss an ice pack in your underwear, and *voilà!* Good as new. A little pro tip I also learned was to take some baby diapers or feminine hygiene pads and put them in the freezer before your baby is born. When you get home and you no longer have those convenient bags of ice from the hospital, you can just pull one of those suckers out of the freezer and use it.

# CHAPTER 3

# PREGNANCY

Let's talk about the elephant in the room, and no, I do not mean you! Pregnancy is a beautiful thing when you think about it: you are creating a whole human being inside of you. But it is not always sunshine and fairy tales. Sometimes pregnancy includes unshaved legs, swollen feet, peeing your pants, and acne . . . yes, acne. Thank you to all the people who failed to mention that I would look like a teenage boy during pregnancy! As if being fat and uncomfortable were not bad enough.

Most pregnant women have been there: You are on your fifth donut, you have not washed your hair, and could not reach your legs even if you wanted to shave them. With a mouthful of donut, you look up and see another pregnant lady who looks like she just stepped off the red carpet. You look down at your wrinkled, stained shirt and secretly compare yourself to this woman, someone who manages to make pregnancy look like a beauty contest. If you have not experienced this feeling, you are probably the woman the rest of us are comparing ourselves to! (Just kidding, because she has been there too.)

But let's not get caught up in the negatives. There are so many positives to pregnancy. One major thing is that your libido skyrockets, which is a plus for both you and hubby. Around your second trimester, the blood flow to your genitals starts to increase, your vagina starts creating more lubrication, and your clitoris becomes more sensitive. Add these all together and you have yourself the makings of an enjoyable sex life! Enjoy it while it lasts and make the most of your hyper sex drive; not only will it help your pregnancy-induced hormonal roller coaster, but it'll also have your spouse enjoying this pregnancy thing too.

Wait . . . hormonal roller coaster? As your body changes, so will your moods! Mood swings are a common occurrence during pregnancy as your body adjusts to the new hormones coursing through your system. Give yourself some grace as you ride the pregnancy hormone roller coaster. Whether you experience an increase of estrogen from your female embryo, or progesterone from your male embryo, or you are just stressed about this new life you are creating and what it means for your future, know that you are not alone.

I will tell you a secret, but you must promise not to share it! Before children, I never produced much estrogen; my progesterone levels were always high and got even higher each time I got pregnant with another boy. By the time I got pregnant with a little girl, the introduction of estrogen was a shock to my body. I went from feeling in control of my emotions and generally standoffish to constantly emotional and moody. The more my baby grew—and more and more estrogen began coursing through my veins—the less I was able to control my emotions (and my bladder).

One day in my eighth month of pregnancy, after a ridiculously hard day at work, my two sons pushed me when I was already at the end of the rope—a rope that was much shorter thanks to my final trimester of pregnancy. Obviously, whatever happened was something minute and trivial, as today I can't even remember what set me off. But at the time? It was catastrophic. There I was yelling, crying . . . and peeing . . . as my kids stood there in shock. They watched me throw a full blown two-year-old tantrum, and I was in my thirties. I stomped off, pee running down my leg, screaming and crying all the way down the hall. The story is hilarious now, but at the time I was at the end of my emotional rope and did not know how to deal with those feelings or express them in a healthy way.

Mood swings are not something you can avoid during pregnancy; in fact, they are one of the things you can expect to have and for which you can try to prepare. However, no matter how much you mentally prepare yourself for the hormones to hit, one cannot fully prepare themselves. So, when they do hit, there are a few things you can do so you don't end up stomping down the hallway, leaving a trail of urine. First off, give yourself a lot of grace (I know, I keep saying that): you may be acting like a crazy person, but you are literally *making* a human. Make sure your spouse or the people close to you know that you are dealing with pregnancy hormones and how they can help. Make room in your schedule for naps; sleeping isn't always easy when you are expecting, and a lack of sleep can add to your already increased stress levels. Believe it or not, but your diet during pregnancy is a huge contributor to the crazy hormones. Eating enough protein and healthy fats while avoiding junk food can really help balance your mood and your pregnancy brain!

Have you ever heard of "baby brain" or pregnancy brain? Well, I am here to tell you that this is a real thing, and it is all thanks to the hormones and sleep issues we just talked about. You are rocking along through your pregnancy when you suddenly start to notice how forgetful you have become or how foggy your brain seems to be. Once you were able to multitask like it was an Olympic sport, but now you are struggling to concentrate on even one task. Look on the bright side: you FINALLY have an excuse for why you don't remember someone's name or forgot to wish them a happy birthday. Now instead of getting annoyed when you forget to do something, people will think it is adorable and endearing. So, live it up, pregnancy is literally the only time in your life where your husband won't leave you if you call him by your ex's name. But do not worry, Mama, things will get back to normal . . . about six months after baby is born.

Pregnancy is more difficult than people make it out to be: it is hard emotionally, physically, and mentally. Don't let yourself or others make you feel like there is something wrong with you because you don't feel birds chirping happily during every second of your pregnancy. I felt like I always needed to be happy; if I was not, I worried I was doing an injustice to the unborn child I was carrying in my womb. Other well-meaning moms would tell me that my child would be able to feel my bad moods and negativity; they said this could affect the baby's development. Instead of ignoring their well-intentioned misinformation, I made my life and the lives of those around me miserable trying to always be positive. You don't need to pretend to feel one way when you actually feel another. What you do need to do is take care of yourself—body, mind, and soul. If I could give an expectant mother one shred of advice, it would be to take care of yourself in every way you can: eat that cookie, take that bath, have a good cry. Whatever it takes, take care of you.

## PHYSICAL SURPRISES

Some of the pregnancy symptoms I've mentioned are commonly known (but definitely still worth talking about) and some are less common or less talked about. Yet the unknown symptoms rear their heads whether we know about them or not, and I always wanted to know what could happen. I felt better when I knew something I'd experienced had happened to other moms too, and the advice of someone who has firsthand experience is the best advice. So here are some other situations you may find yourself in, along with the best advice I could source for each issue.

Your belly will itch like a mother trucker in your final trimester.

—Kaitlan

Although many mamas will tell you that itching is common throughout your whole pregnancy (this is thanks to the hormones), that final trimester is especially itchy as your body stretches to accommodate your growing baby. Putting lotion on daily, from the very beginning of your pregnancy, will help with the itching at the end and will help with stretch marks!

Precursor for the next few sentences. If you love your stretchmarks and just hate the idea of not having them . . . skip the next few paragraphs and move to the next one.

When it comes to stretch marks, I am probably the worst person to be handing out advice because I *don't* want them! I guess that makes me a bad mom, but so be it. I just want to be able to bring a child into this earth without walking around with stretch marks for the rest of my life like some kind of sign advertising that I have given birth. Trust me, the douple shot of espresso in my hand, the kids hanging off me, and the way

I talk to people easily tips people off that I am a mom. I don't need physical marks to prove it! If you are like me and want the experience of having babies without the physical proof, then you will want to read the next paragraph!

I don't know about you, but for me, the moment I found out I was pregnant I felt like I could finally stop sucking in and actually enjoy unhealthy foods without the fear of getting fat. However, pregnant or not, those unhealthy foods and weight gain contribute to stretch marks. Gaining too much weight during pregnancy and an unhealthy diet can also lead to gestational diabetes. My main suggestion on how to prevent both of these effects is to put down the donut and sub it with a nice salad. That salad also helps prevent stretch marks, as do many other nutrient-rich foods (like salmon or dark chocolate). Make sure you are taking a daily prenatal vitamin and include food in your diet that is high in vitamin C (like broccoli, oranges, or strawberries).

Now for the fun stuff! Apply vitamin E oil and/or lotion to your belly daily from the moment you find out that you're pregnant. If you wait until the stretch marks are forming before you start putting lotion on, you will be too late and will most likely have your own set of tiger stripes. StretcHeal is my personal recommendation, but you can only purchase it on their website. Mama Mia's Goodbye Stretch Marks is another great one, but tends to be on the more expensive side. Palmers' coconut oil stretch mark lotion can be purchased at any Walmart or drug store and tends to fit everybody's budget. Whatever you chose to use, just make sure you are not using it sparingly: lather it on as often as you can for the duration of your pregnancy. In the end, you will be left with few to no stretchmarks and healthier skin that is more prone to regain its original prebirth shape.

> Nobody mentioned losing my mucus plug, or I just did not read far enough into my books. But there it was, floating in the toilet bowl! Scared me. FYI this is normal. And the stretch marks hit right before giving birth. I was so sure I had dodged that bullet.
>
> —Ashley

This particular topic is a serious pet peeve of mine. Women have been giving birth for thousands of years, and for thousands of years they have had to lose their mucus plug. So why on earth have ob-gyn's not figured out that they need to tell their first-time moms that this is going to happen, so they don't freak out thinking something bad is happening? This is probably the main question I see on pregnancy pages. "What is this?" "Do I need to go to the hospital?" "I wiped and this weird stuff was on the paper . . ." The questions go on and on. I want to make sure my readers know what this is, so that when you lose your plug you are prepared.

Throughout your pregnancy your body produces mucus, which forms a barrier at the base of your cervical canal. This barrier prevents things from entering your uterus and keeps that area moist and protected. As your body begins to prepare for the birth of your baby, your cervix softens and that mucus plugs falls out. We refer to that process as "losing your mucus plug." This is a perfectly natural process and is indeed great news; it means that the birth of your new baby is coming soon! (Keep in mind that *soon* is a relative term.) So don't be surprised when you look in the toilet and see a huge booger floating in the water, or wipe and see the same thing on your toilet paper. This is a natural process that takes place as your body prepares for birth.

> Insomnia hits in the last few weeks. Maybe it is your body getting used to baby? Whatever it is, you cannot sleep—and every time you wake up, you must pee, and it is *impossible* to get out of bed. I conceded to sleeping in a chair since it was easier to get out of when I needed to pee forty-seven times a night.
>
> —Emma

This comment from Emma makes me giggle. I remember those last few nights after I hit week thirty-five (thank goodness all my babies were early), when I just couldn't fall asleep to save my life. Rolling over after thirty-five weeks of pregnancy should seriously be an Olympic sport. It takes everything you have to get that big ole whale body flopped over. Then you are wide awake again . . . and of course, since you are awake, you have to pee. You wait it out until you are certain you will wet the bed. You heave-ho, grunt a fart out, twist and turn until somehow you manage to get out of bed. You're off to the bathroom as you squeeze your legs together, begging God to keep you from wetting your pants. You sit down and . . . one drop comes out. Awesome. You can thank baby for that pressure in your bladder that causes you to feel the constant need to pee. This late in your final trimester, baby is now head down in the birthing canal, getting ready for the big debut. Now it is off to bed again where it takes forty-seven different positions, three fans, thirty pillows, and a sacrifice to the gods for you to fall back asleep.

> In the beginning, the nausea and change in hormones was intense. People forgot to mention that the nausea comes back towards the end of your pregnancy.
>
> —Leandra

> I threw up *a lot*, even water. I lost weight and looked sickly and thin, but I hated how I felt. I was so miserable.
>
> —Emily

Nausea . . . morning sickness . . . gravidarum . . . whatever you want to call it, it sucks. For some women, it is how they can tell they are pregnant, other women never experience it, and some live with an extreme version called hyperemesis gravidarum (discussed later in this chapter). There is no rhyme or reason as to why some people get morning sickness and others don't, when it hits or if it will. For my first son it was all-day sickness; I couldn't understand why anyone would call it *morning* sickness when it literally lasted from the moment I woke up to the moment I went to bed. At least with him, it finished as quickly as it had started. My second son was the same, except my morning sickness was more like afternoon sickness. By my third son, I think my body had gotten used to it because there was no morning sickness, just a lot of naps.

By the time my daughter came along eight years later, my body had apparently forgotten what to do in pregnancy, so for the first three months I battled hellacious morning sickness. I had the opportunity to travel to Ireland while in my first trimester (something I do not recommend). The flight was twelve hours of praying that I wouldn't vomit on the sweet kid sitting next to me, trying to force myself to stay asleep and crying because I was certain everybody was about to see and smell what I just had for lunch. Because I traveled alone, I booked sightseeing tours so that I wouldn't have to attempt to drive my manual car in the opposite direction without the use of my GPS to tell me where to go (also something I don't recommend). I had to sit at the front of the bus, which sometimes meant asking the person already sitting there to move, then sleeping the whole trip for the same reasons as on the plane.

In the United States, your ob-gyn can prescribe a suppository to help with the nausea and vomiting, but in Ireland the solution was all things ginger, such as ginger ale and ginger candy. There are other natural methods that have helped women in the past if you don't feel up to having something shoved up your bum and ginger isn't your thing. Saltine crackers and sprite first thing in the morning before getting out of bed can help, as can sucking on peppermint candies throughout the day. Instead of eating large meals, eat small snacks every two hours or so, and drink lots and lots of water. Avoid nausea triggers. For me, that meant steering clear of seafood and truffle fries. Sounds stupid, but for me, carrying around a lemon helped offset those smells that might trigger my nausea. Ultimately, find what works for you and stick with it until that pesky nausea goes away (usually after the first trimester).

> Heartburn . . . oh, the heartburn. By the way, my baby came out with *tons* of hair, just like the old wives' tale says.
>
> **—Melissa**

Have you ever heard the old wives' tale that states if you have heartburn during pregnancy your baby will come out with a full head of hair? Most people still swear by it, but I may have to debunk that one. My heartburn was the worst with my daughter, and she came out as bald as a puppy. That is just one of many old wives' tales that pertain to pregnancy, such as "If you have severe morning sickness, you are having a girl" and "Craving salty foods means you are having a boy." However, I craved donuts and ice cream with two of my sons, so I'm not sure how well that last one holds up.

If you enjoy having a little fun during your pregnancy and don't care about what sex you are having, I recommend googling old wives' tales and seeing how many you can try and what they predict. I tried nearly a dozen different old wives' tales to find out the sex of my first baby and every single one of them said I was having a girl. So, imagine my disappointment when the doctors pointed out his penis on the ultrasound screen. I learned my lesson and didn't try any of those same tests with my other kids; I didn't want to get excited about a certain sex and then experience the letdown when it wasn't right.

> Nobody told me I would crave food I hate. I ate so many freaking jalapenos.
>
> **—Amanda**

While I was pregnant with my son, I craved cheese and salad topping sandwiches. I must have had one every day. After giving birth, I made one . . . it was the most disgusting thing I had ever eaten. Still not as bad as my sister though. She craved sardines and cherry pie filling (gag).

—Tonya

We've all heard the stories of strange cravings during pregnancy. I can only confirm the truth behind these stories. No matter what strange thing you've heard of (or craved yourself), there's probably something even stranger out there: sardines with mustard sauce, chocolate on pizza, ice cream with cold chicken, cupcakes with bacon, and apples with salt and vinegar. Now, not every craving is some disgusting combination of foods that don't belong together. Some cravings are simpler, like chocolate ice cream when you normally despise chocolate, generic brand cereal, mangoes, or donuts. Women crave so many funny (and often absolutely disgusting) things while pregnant, but who cares! If it makes mama happy, then go for it! Then for fun after you deliver, try that chocolate on pizza concoction that you couldn't get enough of during pregnancy, and see if you still like it!

I do not care how you divide forty weeks; it still equals ten months!

—Michelle

> Thirty-seven weeks is still considered "full term." With my second, I went into labor . . . but was in denial about being in labor. We had a planned, home birth. I was literally saying, "I'm not in labor, he's too early at thirty-seven weeks," all the way until fifteen minutes before he showed up, a full seven pounds.
>
> —Jaklin

All of my babies were born at thirty-six weeks and were considered full-term babies. At your thirty-six-week appointment your doctor will give you the green light and let you know that it is now officially "safe" to have baby. By this time, they are no longer considered a preemie, but rather full term.

## HYPEREMESIS GRAVIDARUM
*Contributed by Ayron D.*

Most people do not know what this is, but I do, and it is a nightmare. It is morning sickness twenty-four hours a day, seven days a week, for nine months. It is not just queasiness: It's vomiting up to twenty times a day and dry heaving in between. It is throwing up so hard you pop blood vessels all over your face, neck, and chest. It is not being able to get up to take care of your older children. It is relying on your husband to get both you and the kids situated in the morning before he heads off to work because you will not be able to do anything.

Hyperemesis gravidarum is being carried to the car when you need to go to the hospital for fluids, and going so often that you have blown veins all over your arms and wind up looking like a junkie. It is knowing the hospital staff by name because you are there nearly every day. It is losing weight as opposed to gaining weight during pregnancy and begging God not to let you or your baby die. It is needles, pumps, and medications that are supposed to stave off the vomiting, if even for a few minutes. It is your husband waking you up every two hours to give you a sip of Gatorade, and then saving the bottles to use as sharps containers.

Hyperemesis gravidarum is having your husband carry you down the stairs because you are too weak to walk. It is accepting help in the shower because you cannot stand and wash your hair at the same time. It is bruises all over your swollen belly from your pumps and needle sites. It is rashes from the adhesives they use to lock down your IV. It is begging your doctor for a bolus because the meds are not working today. It is being told by well-meaning people that you just need to eat saltines before getting out of bed because they don't understand that you are liable to choke on them when they are coming back up because they are so dry. It is learning that peanut butter and grilled cheese have a better chance of staying down and learning that soft-serve ice cream or Kool-Aid are easiest coming back up. It is learning that throwing up coffee is terrible and vomiting up your favorite foods may lead to a lifelong aversion to them.

It is understandable that pregnancy is not beautiful or full of joy when all you can think about is how you are going to make it to the end without dying. When experiencing hyperemesis gravidarum, even the most levelheaded women may contemplate abortion or suicide just to end the misery.

You wake up each morning praying that the day will be a "fluffy day." Those days are like a light in the middle of the darkest tunnel. You can eat on those days and not throw up nearly as much. You know you are experiencing a fluffy day when, after weeks of not being able to bear even the thought of food, you will suddenly have cravings.

If you experience this condition, know that you are not alone. If you somebody you love is going through this, understand how hard it is and be there for them. Keep the well-meaning advice to yourself and learn how to pray for them and care for them.

# CHAPTER 4

# IS IT LABOR OR BAD FOOD?

There is no exact methodology when it comes to stimulating contractions or provoking labor, just like there are no exact symptoms that tell you for sure that you are in labor. Different tricks to stimulate labor work differently for every woman, and pre-labor and labor symptoms will also vary from person to person. Sometimes it's hard to know if you're experiencing labor, false labor, indigestion, or plain and simple nerves. In this chapter, I'll share what I know from my own experience as well as tips and insights from other women. Just remember: do not do anything to stimulate labor until your ob-gyn has given you the green light!

## SIGNS OF POSSIBLE LABOR

Let's start with a small disclaimer: although I am a medical professional and worked in this field, I am not providing medical advice. My advice is from the perspective of a mom who has experienced multiple pregnancies and births. I couple my personal experiences and those of other mamas to provide anecdotal information and advice that I hope you find helpful. All of this information is sourced from my own experience and from

51

people I know and trust, but of course you should always consult your doctor, midwife, or other medical professional if you have additional questions. Under no circumstances do I recommend you take the advice of your friends over that of your ob-gyn.

With that said, let's look at a few signs that might hint your body is telling you labor is close:

- Back pain or pressure that is constant and does not go away with your usual tricks
- Swelling in the ankles and vagina
- Loss of the mucous plug. As we discussed in chapter 3, this looks like you peed out a snail and it could be slightly bloody.
- Your water breaks—not to be mistaken for when the baby kicks you and you tinkle
- Nesting—a sudden urge to clean, organize, etc.
- Fatigue *or* a sudden increase of energy
- Your belly looks and feels lower
- Hard(er) time sleeping
- Pressure in between your legs—a sensation like you could reach up and feel the baby's head popping out (I seriously felt like my vagina was on the floor)
- Diarrhea
- Your baby is less active
- Period-like cramps

## BRAXTON-HICKS

Have you ever had a friend that told you that she was having contractions but not to worry, it was just Braxton-Hicks? Or you are watching a movie and the character goes to the hospital only to leave a short time later due to "false labor"? What is false labor or Braxton-Hicks? To understand what false labor is, let's go back to the conversation about the mucus plug. You lose your mucus plug as your cervix is softening for labor. Well, at the same time that your cervix is softening, it also thins and begins practicing for the real event. Braxton-Hicks are sporadic "practice" contractions that last anywhere from a few seconds to a few minutes and feel like menstrual cramps.

These practice contractions can happen at any point during your second and third trimester, especially if you have been particularly active or if you have partaken in a "romantic rendezvous" with your significant other (by "rendezvous" I mean *sex*). You will know they are Braxton-Hicks because of their irregular patterns, the ability to make them stop, and their lack of intensity. No hospital or ob-gyn will fault you for getting checked out when you feel these contractions, but you can avoid an unnecessary trip to Labor and Delivery (L&D for short) by drinking a large glass of water and laying on your left side. If the contractions go away, it was false labor. If the contractions become more consistent, then it is most likely actual labor.

## TIPS FOR ENCOURAGING HEALTHY LABOR

Maybe you're on baby three or four and you know what I mean, or maybe this is baby number one for you, and you haven't gotten there yet . . . but many mamas will agree, there comes a time when you're ready for the little one to be out! This comes from someone that *loved* every single second of being pregnant. I have even considered surrogacy because I love the pregnancy process so much. However, even I get to the point that I am just flat done . . . or should I say "round" done? Once you hit week thirty-six and you have been given the all-clear from your ob-gyn, you can start the eviction process for your little one. The recommendations listed below were given to me by my ob-gyn, and it is safe to assume your ob-gyn will offer up some of these same options if you ask.

**Tip #1: Sex**
This is a fun one. Let's hear from some women who have found this option successful for getting baby on the move. I can't say that this worked for me, but I definitely tried! Although I do know many women who swear by this method . . . either way, it's worth the try for me! Dad may not mind the sudden change in arousal, although most guys don't like having sex in the final trimester—apparently, they are afraid they will feel the baby while they are in there!

> I had sex the night after my OB appointment (at her recommendation). My water broke during sex!
> —Mary

> According to my doctor, orgasming may help stimulate the uterus. Sex can trigger the release of oxytocin, and semen contains prostaglandins which can help ripen the cervix. Not guaranteed, but it is worth a shot!
> —Stephanie

**Tip #2: Walking and Squats**

Although I can say with certainty that neither squatting nor walking put me into labor, I will gladly argue that it was the squatting that made my labors so easy. Not only did I do a lot of walking and squatting in the weeks leading up to my babies' births, but I also did them while I was in labor. I cannot think of a single negative result from walking during pregnancy; not only does it make you feel better, but it also reduces your chance of complications during labor! While in labor, walking helps to reduce labor-induced back aches and labor pains. Squatting helps your hips shift into the best placement for baby to come out, and squatting during contractions makes the process go a little more smoothly and quickly. Squatting during labor is so beneficial that some moms even choose to give birth in a squatted position!

Squatting and walking put me into labor both times.
—Esteffania

Both nights before I went into labor, I did deep squats, nipple stimulation, had my hubby rub my ankles, and we had sex. I went into labor the next day both times.

—Kylee

**Tip #3: Pay Attention to Your Bowels**

Alright, time for a big word: prostaglandins. What in the world are prostaglandins? I am glad you asked! Prostaglandins are the hormones that your body begins to produce in excess to stimulate labor. This may not be something everyone wants to talk about all the time, but it's important to pay attention to what's going on inside you, especially when you know baby may be on her way any minute now. I mean seriously, could you imagine announcing that you are expecting, and someone replies with, "Great! Just remember that diarrhea equals labor." You'd be thinking, *Wtf?* However, it is absolutely true: diarrhea does equal labor. Prostaglandins cause loose stools, and it is believed that you have diarrhea in the days/hours leading up to labor as a way for your body to "clean house" and give your uterus plenty of space to contract during labor.

> I had my baby at thirty-seven weeks. I had irregular Braxton-Hicks for two weeks before they became steady contractions. I had diarrhea the night before I lost my mucus plug and my water broke.
>
> —Leah

> I had diarrhea and lightning crotch (a pregnancy term for sharp vaginal or rectal pain) a week before each of my three deliveries. Those two symptoms are how I knew I was close with each baby.
>
> —Sari

I had a ton of pelvic pain and stomach pain the day before I had my baby.

—Desiree

I had vaginal and rectal pressure like nobody's business in the days leading up to labor. Seriously, I thought she might fall out my bum at any moment.

—Amy

# CHAPTER 5

# PACKING FOR THE HOSPITAL

Packing for the hospital varies for each mama. It may mean grabbing your purse as you head out the door, or it may mean packing like you'll be gone for a month. To better help you determine what you need for your stay at the hospital, here's a checklist of must-haves I've created based off a survey of two hundred women.

While this list is intended to help you think about everything you may want to have with you during a hospital stay, it is important to understand that your needs vary depending on your delivery and the length of your stint in the hospital. For instance, you may walk into Labor and Delivery in the early morning hours, have a quick and complication-free delivery, and be out of there by the next morning. Or you can labor for forty-eight hours, push for three, and then end up having a c-section and find yourself in the hospital for close to a week. Your stay at the hospital all depends on how you and baby did during labor and if there were any complications.

When Kenny was born, I had preeclampsia, which meant I had dangerously high blood pressure and had to be induced. Well, the first thing I learned is that you are *not* a priority when being induced (presumably because . . . well . . . you are not in labor). I went to the doctor that day and was immediately sent to

L&D for an emergency induction. However, when we got there, we learned that L&D was filled to the brim with women *actually* in labor. They literally did not have space for anyone else, in active labor or otherwise. So, the L&D staff monitored my blood pressure and my sons' vitals from a bed they stole from another floor that they hid in the back corner of the waiting room to provide some semblance of privacy.

The staff waited eight hours to start my Pitocin (a medication that stimulates labor), and I was due to have the Pitocin drip for nine hours. Seventeen hours into my stay at the hospital, I finally went into labor and labored for three hours. Once it was time to push, I spent an hour pushing before my doctor decided to assist me and began using different medical (and not-so-medical) devices to help me get my son out. When the suction cup didn't work, my OB pulled out a pair of salad tongs and helped pull Kenny out with my next contraction. Finally, twenty-one hours after arriving at the hospital, I gave birth to a fat little cherub. I had to stay in the hospital for three days after my son's birth because I had lost so much blood thanks to my prolonged pushing and his fat little head. Start to finish, I was in the hospital for four days.

When I went into labor with son number two, I got to the hospital just in time to start pushing. Twenty minutes after arriving at L&D, I gave birth to a perfectly healthy little Malibu Barbie (as the ob-gyn called him). I was released the next morning, less than twelve hours after arriving. My third son would have been just as quick, had the doctors not needed to slow down my labor. They had not received the results of my Group B Strep (GBS) test, and that is something that doctors need in order to determine whether mom needs antibiotics during delivery. Because of that, they slowed my labor down for four hours until I got my negative results. All in all, I was at the hospital for roughly twenty-four hours.

I went into labor on a Sunday night with my daughter, or at least that was when I started having contractions. I called my mom and let her know I may or may not be calling her later because we had spent way too long at Six Flags . . . and I was now having intense contractions. The next morning I woke up feeling like I had been hit by a truck, but oddly enough there were no contractions. I went to see my ob-gyn, who sent me straight to the hospital to be induced, but by that time I was already having contractions again. I checked into L&D on a Monday morning and did not give birth until Wednesday morning, despite forty-eight hours of intense labor. Overall, I spent five days in the hospital. I say all of this just to make one point: it doesn't matter if this is your first or fifth baby, you never know what to expect. I recommend packing as though you are going to be there for a week, and if you spend less time there, great! But if you don't, you are at least prepared.

As a side note: GBS is a bacteria found in all our bodies, and although it does not cause issues for us, it may cause issues to your baby as you deliver them if you don't not receive anti-biotics. All moms get tested for GBS between weeks thirty-five and thirty-seven, and the hospitals receive the results so they can prepare accordingly.

## LIST: FOR MOM

- A "going home" outfit for mom: Trust me, you won't want to go home in the same outfit you arrived in (much less in the hospital gown they provide you) nor will you automatically fit into your pre-pregnancy clothes.

- Hair ties: Let's be real, the last thing you want is your hair getting in your face and in your way when you are in labor.
- Nursing bra: Nursing bras are like that well-kept secret that nobody mentions, but they are absolutely the difference between an enjoyable breastfeeding experience and just about ripping your bra off trying to find your nipple.
- Socks and slippers: You are required to wear nonslip socks at the hospital and trust me, they don't invest in high quality or fashionable socks. Hence the recommendation to bring your own.
- Nursing pads: Typically you are just producing colostrum in the first few days after your baby is born, but you want nursing pads handy when your milk finally drops. Otherwise, the whole world will see that your milk has come in, thanks to the big wet stains on your shirt.
- Comfortable pillow: I was fine with the hospital pillows, but some people can only sleep with their own pillow.
- Robe: Again, not something I used, but I am not the most modest person. I was fine getting up to go to the bathroom or shower with my bum hanging out of my sexy hospital gown, but some women prefer to cover up a bit more.
- Shower flip flops: This is another personal decision. If you are someone that likes to wear flipflops in public showers, you will want to bring them to the hospital. They also recommend you bring them, but it isn't required by any means.
- Makeup and lip balm: ChapStick to me is like a cellphone for a millennial. I *have* to have my ChapStick, and believe me, your lips get chapped during labor. I recommend you bring makeup in case you feel up to taking pics with baby and don't want to look like someone that Jesus brought back to life.

- Adult diapers (Depends): In the hospital, they will provide you with what they call "Victoria secret panties," which are basically cheesecloth-type material boy shorts and the world's largest pad. It is uncomfortable, and the panties don't stay up well, but they do the trick if you haven't learned the secret about adult diapers!
- Essential toiletries
- Snacks
- Lotion
- Phone Charger: Once again, you could be at the hospital for ten hours or ten days; best to be prepared and bring a charger.

> I did not realize when they say pack a bag for the hospital stay that you do not pack your "normal" clothes. There I was with a pair of size two jeans trying to squeeze into them to go home. I ended up wearing the same pants home I wore in.
>
> —Peggy

> I packed jeans for pictures in the hospital. I had a scheduled C-section. I did get them on, but I had to put on two spanks tops beforehand. (The jeans were a size ten; I was a six pre-pregnancy.) Everyone thought I was nuts. The photographer. My doctor. Everyone. I was in fact nuts for doing this.
>
> —Melissa

> Yoga pants or leggings are ideal for going home in.
> —Jessica

If you haven't picked up on what all these people are putting down, let me clarify: leave the jeans at home. Leggings or sweats are the way to go. I may only be thirty-something years old, but I am pretty sure I was an eighty-year-old Hawaiian lady in a past life, because I *love* muumuus. I have always worn muumuus home from the hospital and I have never once regretted my decision. You have either just pushed a watermelon out of your vagina or were cut open with your guts sitting on your stomach—the last thing you want to do is try to fight with a pair of pants. Your only concern when deciding what to wear home should be what is easy and comfortable.

# LIST: FOR BABY

- Pacifier: Some hospital nursing staff will gladly offer up a pacifier, others will quite literally argue with you over your decision to use one and will refuse to give you a pacifier. Either way, bringing your own is a good idea. If the hospital does provide one, it will be the green Avent soothie pacifier, so I recommend bringing a pacifier with a different nipple type in case your baby doesn't like the soothie.
- Car seat: You will not be able to leave the hospital without baby safely strapped into their car seat.
- A "going home" outfit for baby: I recommend bringing a preemie, newborn, and zero to three month outfit, that way

no matter how big or small he is, you will have something that fits him.

- Boppy: I personally recommend bringing your Boppy just because it makes life so much easier when nursing and holding your baby.

# LIST: FOR DAD

- Blanket: The hospital may or may not have enough blankets to provide dad with one and his comfort is just as important as yours.
- Underwear
- Pillow: Same concept as the blanket, the hospital may not have extra pillows for dad.
- Laptop, phone, charger(s), camera, etc.

When you pack a bag, put a couple of clean pairs of underwear in for hubby too. Being induced does not guarantee a quick delivery.

—Dana

Bring a pillow and blanket for Dad, something for him to do, and an extra-long charger too. He will have a lot of down time while you are in labor, so you have two choices: have him hover or give him something to do!

—Chelle

When you pack your bag include everything! Shampoo, soap—everything. I did not anticipate a C-section and ended up at the hospital longer than I thought.

—Ashley

# CHAPTER 6

# YOU TRY PUSHING OUT A WATERMELON!

I feel like this: once you have pushed four children out of you, you can call yourself some type of expert. You may not have gone to school to learn about the birthing process, but by baby number four, you are bound to have learned something. And yet, you have also learned nothing. Every time is different. No matter how many times you give birth, each birth is unique. To give you an idea of just how different each birth can be, in this chapter I will walk you through each of my four births.

## BABY #1

During my first pregnancy, I read every book I could get my hands on and attended every class available to me. I was determined to go into the birthing process completely educated and prepared. Yeah . . . that did not happen.

My pregnancy was just dandy for the first six months. I hit every milestone as I was supposed to and was feeling great as I entered my final trimester. But it seemed to all go downhill once I hit my final three months.

The first shocking realization occurred during lunch as I was eating my favorite fruit. As my lips and throat began to swell, I realized I was having an allergic reaction to a fruit I had eaten dozens of times. The doctors in the emergency room informed me that throughout pregnancy, not only does your body change, but your sensitivities do as well. For me, those changes in sensitivity meant a newfound allergy to pitted fruits.

My third trimester adventures did not end there. A few weeks later, I was put on bedrest after going into preterm labor. I had called my ob-gyn after a day of what I believed were Braxton-Hicks (the "practice" contractions that occur before true labor) to see what I could do to make them subside. She recommended I drink a big glass of water and lie on my left side. If the contractions did not go away, she informed me they may be real contractions. Sure enough, they did not go away. I found myself in pre-term labor at just thirty weeks. I went to the hospital where they gave me medications to stop the labor and sent me home, on bedrest, for the next six weeks until my son was deemed full term.

At thirty-six weeks, I went in for my weekly doctor's appointment. They found indicators of preeclampsia (the onset of high blood pressure and protein in your urine). After the doctors tried unsuccessfully to lower my dangerously high blood pressure, I was whisked off to Labor and Delivery to be induced. My doctors had estimated my son's weight to be around six pounds and determined it was safe for me to have him. Let me tell you something: if you can bypass being induced . . . do it.

When you are induced, you are confined to bed as they pump medication into you that will stimulate labor. I did not realize how agonizing laboring in bed was until my second child came along and I had something else with which to compare it. During my second birth, I was able to move around during labor and realized how much of a difference this made. When it came time to deliver my first son, I was so afraid to tear that I insisted my doctor do an episiotomy if it even appeared I might tear. But as it turns out, when you tear naturally during vaginal birth it heals more easily and is not as painful after the birth. I sure wish someone had told me that. I couldn't sit up straight for a month after my son was born because of the surgical incision I has insisted upon.

> Do not get an episiotomy unless necessary. Some doctors are in a hurry and are not nice about them.
> —Elizabeth

My son was born a fat and healthy eight pounds, one ounce. His weight was the first indication that weight guessing prior to birth is just that—guessing! After my baby was out, my doctor told me that had my little boy been an ounce bigger I would not have been able to push him out, and trust me, my body felt every one of his ounces. I was not able to hold my son without assistance for the first few days because I was anemic from the amount of blood I had lost during labor, and I couldn't get up unless a nurse was there to assist me. I felt depressed and helpless because nobody had told me that these things could happen during labor.

Because I was anemic, they kept me in the hospital a few days longer than normal to ensure my blood count came back up and I would not need a transfusion. Being in the hospital is somewhere between being in a hotel with room service and being tortured by terrorists. On the one hand, I was waited on hand and foot. If I needed food, I just called a number and whatever I wanted was delivered to my bedside. My bed linens were changed daily, and I was never without a refreshing beverage. On the other hand, it was impossible to sleep when nurses and doctors were in my room every thirty minutes insisting on "massaging" my extremely sore uterus to ensure it was shrinking or checking my vital signs. Then, the moment I got my brand-new crying baby to sleep, a nurse would come in and announce that it was bath time!

I remember going to the bathroom for the first time after birth and being bewildered as to why a nurse was coming in with me. Apparently, she was there to clean up any mess I might make using the restroom, a gesture I appreciated when I stood up off the toilet and a blood clot the size of a basketball fell on the floor. I was humiliated and stood there crying as I stared at it. The very gracious nurse simply said, "Ah, that's why you've been cramping," and gingerly escorted me back to bed so she could go clean it up.

> The nurse will go with you to the bathroom to clean things up . . . I did not know that, and I was like, "I just have to pee, why are you here?"
> —Brenda

When it was time to get discharged, I was terrified and wanted to beg them to let me stay another night. What happened if I got home and had a question and didn't know what to do? What would I do without having the experts just one click away?

Despite my fears and reluctance to go home, they sent us packing, and we were left to figure out the whole parenting thing on our own. I was lucky that I was pregnant at the same time as a good friend so that she and I were able to bounce ideas off one another. I also battled PPD (postpartum depression) thanks to the anemia and inability to hold my son without help that first week, but I was lucky enough to have a mom and husband to support me and help me through it.

# BABY #2

My second son arrived just twenty-two months after the birth of my first son. This time, I was certain I knew what to expect. This time, when I went into labor, I thought I knew exactly what was going on. In case you can't already tell . . . things didn't go quite as I anticipated.

I was already laboring when my mom and I went to the mall to do some shopping, based on the advice given to us by my amazing doula (a type of birthing coach). Her suggestion was to labor at home (or in this case, the mall) for as long as possible before going to the hospital. I would recommend just walking around your neighborhood instead, not so much for you as for the other people at the mall. The sheer fear and panic I saw in people's eyes when they realized I was in labor at the mall was more than a little amusing to me, but definitely not to them. Oh, and I had to fight my contractions as I drove home from the mall.

Two times during this pregnancy, we rushed (prematurely) to the hospital due to my "water breaking." The first time, the doctors informed me that my son had just kicked my bladder a little too hard. That's right—I rushed to the hospital because I had peed my pants! The second time, I was holding my oldest son when I felt warmth between my legs. At first, I thought my son had peed on me. Then I realized my water had broken.

This time, though, my water really had broken! Except . . . it was not the sac with the baby in it. It turned out I had formed two sacks. As my son grew, he eventually ruptured the second sac. I was once again sent home with the assurance that I was not in labor. Because of this, my husband nearly missed his son's birth when I finally did go into labor!

A short time into my actual labor, my doula and I decided we should go to L&D so they could determine how far I had progressed in labor and give us an estimate on how much longer I had. This would help us determine how long to labor at home before returning to the hospital. This decision was more for my peace of mind than my doula's; if it had been up to her, we would have waited longer. I just felt like I needed to go to the hospital, and she was happy to support whatever decisions I made. Here is one thing I have learned from all the time I have spent at the hospital: you will have amazing nurses, and you will have nurses straight out of hell. Please hear me when I say that it is okay to request another nurse when the latter occurs.

The nurse assigned to me when we first went in to check my progress walked into the room, took one look at me, and said disgustedly, "If you were in labor, you wouldn't be laughing. I am going to go get your discharge papers." She then stormed off.

My doula went out and found another nurse and asked her to check my progress, letting her know that we simply wanted to know how far dilated I was so we could estimate how much longer I could labor at home. The nurse kindly obliged and set about checking my progress. She put her fingers in to check my cervix and, looking quite shocked, said "Yeah, you're not in labor. You're having your baby!" By the time the first nurse got back with my discharge papers, I was holding my new son in my arms. The lesson I hope you take from this experience is to not be afraid to ask for a second opinion, and to only trust those who take the time to conduct a thorough exam! Had it not been for that second nurse, I would have had my son in the elevator on our way back to the car.

As a side note, I want to talk to you about doulas. As I mentioned previously, a doula is a type of birthing coach, but they are also much more. A doula is someone who is there for you throughout your entire pregnancy. They help you through all the tough times and they are there to answer any questions you may have during pregnancy and delivery. Most important, a doula can be your voice when you don't have one. Had it not been for my doula, my birthing experience would have been quite different. All I knew to do when the nurse was mean to me was cry, but she hunted down another nurse and made sure they did what they were supposed to do.

Although doulas are not usually healthcare professionals, they have a vast amount of experience and knowledge when it comes to pregnancy, labor, and birth. They are phenomenal to have around when you are a first-time parent or a single parent because they can be that pillar for you to lean on. However, I chose a doula for my second baby because I learned with my first that I needed to have a voice outside of mine in the room. I have never regretted that decision and I honestly don't think you will either.

# BABY #3

No one told me that with each natural labor and natural birth, the kid comes racing out faster and faster each time. By baby #3, I almost had her at home after an amazingly fast two-hour labor.

**—Jannette**

While in my final month of pregnancy with my third son, I woke up early in the morning with the most terrible urge to use the bathroom. I spent nearly thirty minutes in the bathroom trying to have a bowel movement before I realized that what I was feeling was the urge to push. I had been in labor and had not realized it. We rushed to the hospital, where the staff were blasé until I mentioned it was my third child and I felt the urge to push. Apparently, that's all I needed to say. The next thing I knew they were rushing around and all business. I mentioned that I wanted an epidural and was told that I was too far progressed in my labor and that the anesthesiologist had too many people to do before me, so I would be having him all natural—an answer that had me bawling my eyes out. I am not too proud to admit that the only way I got through labor and birth was the beautiful solace of an epidural. The thought of not having one and having to feel every last birthing pain was terrifying.

Luckily for me, my third son wanted to be born before I had been given the results of my strep B test, and that is a big no-no. If I'd had strep B, they would have needed to give me antibiotics for a few hours before my delivery, but they couldn't know until my doctor's office opened four hours later. Suddenly, not only was there time for an epidural, but the anesthesiologist walked in almost immediately. The ob-gyn on duty was hoping that an epidural would slow my labor down long enough to get the results from my doctor and start me on antibiotics just in case. Once my test came back negative, they gave their blessing for my baby to be born and I had him shortly thereafter.

# BABY #4

> My first was twelve hours, second was six hours, and my last one less than three . . . homeboy fell out after one push.
>
> —Jessica

You would think after three children, the fourth one would just walk right out. Push once, then wham-bam-thank-you-ma'am, your baby is born. Before baby number four, my labors had ranged from six hours after being induced to a mere twenty minutes. Why should this baby be any different?

I went into labor after an evening at Six Flags with my sons. I called my mom and let her know I was having bad contractions, but I assumed it was from walking nearly seven miles while out with my kids. I woke up the following morning feeling like I was getting sick, but I no longer had contractions. I went to work, and a short time later I told a colleague that I thought I might be in labor. By the time I got to my ob-gyn's office, I felt like I had been hit by a truck.

After a quick exam, my doctor said, "Let's go have a baby," and told me he would meet me at the hospital. I drove over to the hospital and was admitted around lunch time on Monday afternoon. After hooking me up to the monitors, the nurse told me I was indeed in labor and said the machines were picking up mild contractions. Next they checked my cervix. Sure enough, I was dilated, but barely to two centimeters. By Tuesday morning, I had only progressed to four, despite off-the-chart contractions that had kept me up all night.

Here's what I hope you remember after reading this story: the nurses and doctors may be the professionals, but *you* know your body like no one else does. On Tuesday morning, I was sitting in bed having just had my cervix checked when I felt a warm liquid pooling between my legs. I would have thought my water had broken, except that they had broken my water hours earlier. So I reached down. When I brought my hand up, it was covered in blood and water. I reached down again. This time, I felt the hair on my baby's head. I called out to the nurse, the one who had just checked me, and I insisted that it was time to push.

The nurse laughed, said she had just checked me, and then assured me there was no way I was ready to push. After enough griping, the nurse put on a glove to see where the baby was. Suddenly it was all chaos and running as they tried to get set up before my baby came out. I was squeezing my legs shut as I watched people running around the room desperately trying to get ready. I delivered a healthy little girl three minutes after my doctor arrived . . . after being in labor for over twenty-four hours.

# THE LESS GLAMOROUS MOMENTS

**Inducing**

I have been induced TWICE, and I can tell you, I do not recommend it. It sounds amazing: you go into the hospital not in labor, they put you into labor, and *voilà*! You get to have your baby. But that is not what happens. You are second priority to the women who are *actually* in labor—at least until the Pitocin has done its job and you start to be in active labor, which could be anywhere from a few hours to several days. I understand that some women don't have the option of not being induced (I was one of them), but for the women that can choose to be induced, I recommend you wait until your baby decides to come. Your body labors more easily when it naturally progresses instead of being forced into it.

> Getting induced sucks.
> I went from having contractions every few minutes and not feeling a thing, to contractions back-to-back with a lot of pain.
> —Sam

> It might take four freaking days of labor from the time of induction until the baby comes out.
> —Monika

**Epidurals**

I am not a big fan of talking about controversial topics such as politics or religion, but with epidurals I make an exception. If you haven't gathered from the rest of this book, I am pro epidural. Shoot, I am pro anything that doesn't make me feel the bowling ball pushing its way out of my vagina, but I digress. I have been told and seen other women get told that they are not a "real" mom because they had an epidural and did not give birth naturally. So let me explain something to you: you are a mom whether you give birth naturally, have an epidural, get a C-section, or bring your baby home from an adoption agency. How your child comes into this world does not make you a mom; raising a child is what makes you a mom.

We all have the idea in our head that it will be like in the movies—our water will break, and then we will labor beautifully at home before waltzing into the birthing center, where we will deliver our child naturally while the nursing staff sings kumbaya, and everyone lives happily ever after. Heck, maybe you know someone who has had that experience, but that is not everyone. Sometimes an epidural is the difference between life and death for you or your baby. I am willing to say you are even *more* of a mom for choosing the epidural you didn't want, if it means saving your baby.

With my first son, I had every intention of having an all-natural birth, and my doctor was very honest with me. She told me that if I didn't have an epidural, I would most certainly have a stroke and die during labor. If I wanted to live, there truly was no other option for me. Ashlee, our C-section contributor, had planned her birthing experience down to the number of times she would push (okay, maybe not that specific, but it was close). She knew exactly what she wanted, and she had even written it down so that the nursing staff would know. What she knew she didn't want was an epidural or a C-section. She had been waiting years to have this baby and she wanted to experience every second of it. Ashlee had been in labor for over thirty-six hours when the decision was made to do a C-section. There were no questions, no discussions—just drugs and rushing her to surgery to try to save both her life and the life of her baby.

I say all this to make sure you know that birth does not always (or maybe ever) go as expected. There is no right or wrong way to have a baby. All that matters is that both mom and baby live to see the day they both leave the hospital. If you want to have an epidural, go for it and don't feel ashamed. If you want to do it all naturally, more power to you! Either way, understand that once you go into labor, you need to be flexible. Things change in the blink of an eye, and you cannot always prepare for everything.

> I do not know if it is the epidural or just all the stress of contractions, but you start to uncontrollably shake and it does not stop until baby comes. Which might mean you are shaking for six hours straight.
>
> **—Anonymous**

> Sometimes you must get an epidural even if you do not want one and other times you do not even get there in time to get an epidural and have to go through it naturally.
>
> **—Lis**

While in labor—after getting my epidural—I was shaking so bad, like I was cold. It was uncontrollable and lasted for about two hours!

—Savannah

Nobody told me that the epidural will make your back forever hurt, and sciatic nerve pain does *not* go away!

—Nickie

**In Closing, Snacks**

Let's be real, being hungry is never fun, but being hungry during or after doing something as intense as giving birth? Even less fun. If you are truly unlucky, you will get to L&D between mealtimes or give birth between mealtimes, and the hospital won't have anything outside of graham crackers to offer you. If you bring your own snacks then you don't have to worry about planning your birthing experience around mealtimes, because we all know how that kind of planning works out. (It doesn't.)

Eat a full meal before you go to the hospital or bring snacks! My water broke soon after lunch. I did not give birth until 5:05 a.m. the next morning. I did not get moved to my room until after breakfast was served (around 7:30 a.m. , I think). I had to beg for food and all I got was a cold muffin!

—**Michelle**

# CHAPTER 7

# POSTPARTUM FUN

I was too focused on the birth of my first baby—and too busy ensuring that my baby had ten fingers and toes and other "minor" details like that—to spend much time thinking about what was to come after the birth. So, the postpartum experience (everything that my body and brain did after birth) came as quite a shock to me.

One thing I did not expect was all the bleeding and pain that came *after* my baby was born. As soon as my sweet babe came out and was wrapped up in my arms, the nurses started "massaging" my uterus (as you may recall I mentioned in the last chapter). What it really felt like they were doing was pushing hard on my already sensitive gut with all their body weight. This massage is intended to reduce bleeding or cramping, but I am fairly sure that it doubles as a medieval torture method.

> After you give birth (seriously like two minutes after, then every few hours) they massage your uterus to make sure everything is going back to where it belongs. I would rather give birth again. Is it illegal to punch someone for doing a uterine massage?
>
> —Summer

That said, I also had the "pleasure" of learning what happens when they *don't* massage your uterus properly after birth. About twelve hours after the birth of my first son, I began feeling cramps I could only describe as labor pains. I cried out to my nurses and they tried to massage my belly, but the pain was too much for me to allow for much of a massage. I felt going to the bathroom would help, so I got up to use the toilet . . . but the moment I stood up from the toilet, a clot the size of a basketball fell onto the floor.

I stood there bawling and staring at this clot—the size of the baby I had just had—sure that my body could not sustain life after losing that much blood (this was before I got into the medical field and was still a bit green). The nurse brushed it off and told me that clots were completely normal; she also said that this particular clot was probably the reason for my ongoing cramps. Sure enough, the cramps immediately dissipated, but I was humiliated and wished I had known that things like that happen after birth.

Apart from cramping, bleeding, and clots, there are other physical changes to expect after birth, like hair loss! You know those beautiful, thick, luscious locks you had during your pregnancy? Yeah, those go away once your baby is born. Suddenly you have nine months of built-up hair loss to contend with. In place of the full head of shiny hair you were accustomed to during pregnancy, you are left with this stringy dry stuff that is supposed to pass as hair. But don't worry too much: whatever does not fall out on its own, your baby will pull out.

> Sixteen months postpartum and my thick pregnancy hair is still coming out in clumps.
> —Jolene

Then there is the hormonal drain you have to contend with after giving birth to a female baby. For nine months, your body enjoyed an extra dose of estrogen, but after birthing, suddenly that estrogen in ripped away from you—so your body revolts! This is where the saying "girls steal your beauty" comes from. The glow of your skin is gone, your hair looks like you stole it from the scarecrow in *The Wizard of Oz*, and you suddenly have acne again . . . you know, that stuff you used forty gallons of makeup to hide on prom night. Except that now you are too tired and emotional to care about covering up the acne. All you want is to find a shirt that does not have spit-up stains on it.

I would say it takes about a year for your body to fully recuperate from childbirth, so give yourself some grace and do not expect to look like a supermodel as you're leaving the birthing center. Remember: those celebrity moms have *teams* that make them appear as if they are not about ready to cry or fall asleep.

With a little help from Photoshop and a personal entourage, you too could look that good after birth. But since I assume most of my readers are normal women without an entourage of makeup artists, personal dressers, and photo editors, my best advice for you is to take time for yourself in those first few weeks. In fact, what I highly recommend is that you take a hint from Japan's routine for new moms.

After giving birth in Japan, a new mom goes to stay at her parents' house for at least a month. The point of this is so that mom can rest, recuperate, and bond with her new baby. While she is occupied with healing and bonding, her family members do all the household chores. Some cultures require the new mom goes on vacation for several weeks after birth, but I cannot remember where I saw that.

However, here in the good ole US of A, most of us only get a maximum of eight to ten weeks off, a respite which does not include someone else doing our laundry or making our meals. After that, it's right back to life as we knew it—except now we have a new baby! That period of eight to ten weeks is not even a standard. Not only that, but the United States is the *only* country in the world with as many other privileges that does not also guarantee that new moms will get time off after their baby is born! Some moms go back to work in as little as a *week* after childbirth. I was one of those moms. I could not even sit up straight yet, but I was back at work pretending I had not just pushed a new human out of my body the week before. Contrast this with Finland, where a new parent (regardless of gender or biological parental status) gets 164 days of paid maternity leave. That is nearly five months! And guess what, single moms? You get to take the maternity leave for both parents, which means you get 328 days—nearly one *year*—of paid maternity leave!

Could you imagine how beneficial it would be to have the first year of your new baby's life off so that you could truly focus on bonding?

Finland isn't the only country that cares about its parents. Sweden offers new parents 480 days of maternity leave, which can be split up between mom and dad, but it is at an 80 percent salary rate for Mom and 90 percent for Dad. I don't know about you, but I would take it! Denmark gives new parents a total of 52 weeks for parental leave; the mother is guaranteed 18 of those weeks, dad gets 2, and then the parents get to choose how the other 32 weeks gets split! Belgium gives moms 15 weeks of maternity leave and dads 10 days of paternity leave.

However maternity or paternity leave looks for you and your family, whether your postpartum recovery is a month at your parents' house, a "mom-caution," a couple of weeks off, or just a few days, remember to take moments for yourself. Have your partner take the baby while you go get a pedicure. Call up a friend to come rock baby while you enjoy a bath by yourself or a meal you did not snag out of the panty while trying to find baby formula. There is no single right way of handling the pleasures and stresses of postpartum, it is just what is going to work for you.

I can tell you, as a mom that stayed home with my sons but did not have the option of having an extended maternity leave with my daughter, taking all the time your employer, state or country (depending on where you are) offers is so worth it. The first few months with a new baby are so crucial for bonding and babies change so dramatically that if you blink, you will miss something.

One of the hardest parts about returning to work so soon after my daughter was born was finding the time to pump. My work schedule was so hectic that I couldn't always sneak away every two hours to pump, which meant my milk supply slowly dwindled. By three months post-partum, my milk supply had completely dried up and I had to make the hard decision to stop nursing. I will say as a caveat here that I fully believe in fed is best; I don't care where the milk comes from, albeit I really enjoyed that bonding time I had when it was just the two of us while she nursed.

## POSTPARTUM BLEEDING AND BLOOD CLOTS

> You will pass blood clots the size of small apples for up to a week after birth. The first time it happened, I thought an organ had fallen out of me.
> —Monika

I already mentioned this earlier in the chapter, but the first clot I passed after the birth of my first child was easily the size of a basketball. If you do not know to expect this, it is a truly terrifying experience. This is normal. As your uterus sheds its lining, blood pools in your uterus and forms a clot (thanks to our wonderful clotting factors—otherwise, we would all bleed to death after giving birth). What isn't normal is heavy bleeding following the birth of your baby or large clots after the first week or two. If you experience these symptoms, you definitely want to call your doctor.

As a nurse by profession, this is super embarrassing to admit. My baby was an emergency C-section three weeks before my due date. I never dilated and never went into labor, so I was shocked to see all the postpartum bleeding. Like *shocked*. I guess I figured I would bypass that experience.

—Yajaira

You will bleed for three to six weeks after having your baby, and then start your period about two weeks after that bleeding stops. Plus it will be the worst period of your life.

—Jacquelyn

I contemplated taking this last comment out but ultimately decided against it, and this is why: we are all different. Our bodies react differently to pregnancy and giving birth (well quite frankly, we react differently to *everything*) which means you may bleed the full six weeks, or you may spot for a few days. The amount of blood you lose after having a baby depends on so many different factors that there is no way to standardize it and say "this is how long you will bleed, this is how many clots or what size clots you will pass, and this is when your cycle will start." I did not bleed heavily after any of my kids, but I also do not have heavy menstrual cycles. A period for me lasts three days and I could leave the same pad on all day and never soak through it, so for me a week of postpartum spotting was all my body needed after babies.

I am not a medical professional (well, I am . . . but not *your* medical professional) so what I will leave you with is this: if you feel like the bleeding or clotting you are experiencing is abnormal, *call your doctor*. Do not hesitate to ask questions or call your ob-gyn if you have concerns; they get paid to ensure you feel comfortable with the process. If the pain you feel during your first period or after birth is abnormal and not on par with previous cycles, call your doctor. It is *always* better to be safe rather than sorry. I'd rather feel stupid for seeing my doctor than not see my doctor and wind up in the hospital or dead.

## VAGINAL PAIN

> If you have a vaginal birth, sit in warm water mixed with Epsom salt. It soothes the area, and salt is an anti-bacterial.
> —Fatima

> The hospital provided me with numbing spray for "down there" after a vaginal birth. It was amazing.
> —Erica

Giving birth is not the worst part, because that pain goes away quickly. Then you are left with stitches . . . oh gosh, the stitches. They make for weeks of uncomfortable pee moments.

**—Autumn**

Lightning crotch sucks.
**—Nickie**

I can't help but to laugh at the reference to "lightning crotch," especially thinking about a new parent reading this and thinking, *What in the heck did I get myself into?* Because I love my readers and all new parents, I am going to address all of the above, starting with the stitches. I have talked about stitches and what to do for them in previous chapters, but let me reiterate: ice and lidocaine spray are your best friends after your baby is born. These two things really help soothe the burning you feel if you have had stitches. I cannot say I agree with Epsom salt and warm baths, but I also cannot say not to try it because I haven't. I just think any form of salt would burn on that freshly torn (or cut) skin.

Lightning crotch can happen either during pregnancy or after, and it just refers to those random lightning-like shots of pain you get in your vaginal area. I have no idea why it occurs and really have no recommendations on how to fix it. The zaps you feel are so sporadic and disappear so quickly that by the time you drew a bath or got out ice, they would be gone.

# CONSTIPATION AND HEMORRHOIDS

The non-medical me says that the constipation you experience after the birth of a baby is because you are so terrified to poop with your stitches that you hold it in . . . and therefore make yourself constipated. The medical me says that constipation is caused by hormones, diet, dehydration, and sometimes medications given during labor. The hospital usually sends you home with stool softeners, but I recommend stopping by your local grocery store or pharmacy and picking some up before baby is born just in case they don't. A high fiber diet will also help with the postpartum constipation, so stock up on broccoli and berries! If all else fails, there are always laxatives, but make sure you use these with the guidance of your doctor.

Hemorrhoids . . . oh, hemorrhoids. Birth is supposed to be such a beautiful time, so why are there so many things associated with it that just aren't so . . . beautiful? Let's start with what hemorrhoids are. Hemorrhoids are swollen veins that can bulge and sometimes protrude out of the anus. For moms, the cause is two-fold: the first is the added pressure baby puts on the anus during the last few weeks of pregnancy, and the second is caused by pushing during a vaginal birth. Although hemorrhoids usually go away on their own within a few days, they can be itchy, irritating, and sometimes down-right painful. Let your doctor know if you are experiencing hemorrhoids after giving birth and they can decide if a treatment plan is necessary.

The constipation postpartum. I started giving all my friends care packages with prunes and fruit leather when they had their babies.

—Amy

Start taking MiraLAX as soon as you can. No one mentioned how bad the first poo would be after.

—Amanda

## MORE AFTERBIRTH EFFECTS THEY FORGOT TO MENTION

If I've learned one thing from being a mom, it's that there's always another surprise around the corner. Whether it's something you didn't think would happen to *you* (even if it happens to other people) or it's something you never even thought to look out for . . . your post-baby body will surprise you.

Nobody told me about the night sweats during postpartum. I did not have it with my first son, but seven years later, with my second, I would wake up drenched in sweat every night.

—Jessica

Back pain after the birth of your baby is normal, especially if you get an epidural or a spinal tap. Expect your back to be sore or just plain hurt for weeks or even months after.

—Sarah

One day you will swear you feel the baby kick [inside you] . . . except he is six months old, and you just have a gas bubble.

—Richelle

I am one of those moms who *loved* being pregnant. Seriously. I loved it so much that I have even contemplated being a surrogate, except I would get too attached to the little bugger even if I knew it wasn't biologically mine. One of my favorite things about being pregnant was feeling my sweet little one in there trying out for the Olympics. I would anxiously anticipate the first little flutter and would feel so lost once by baby was born and no longer got to feel my baby kick . . . until one day, I did. I was sitting there holding my new little bundle when all of a sudden, I felt what I could have *sworn* was a baby kicking me. If I hadn't been holding my baby in my arms, I would have been convinced that he or she was still inside me.

It turns out those phantom baby kicks are normal and to be expected after having a baby. They even have a cool name for those feelings—they're called *phantom kicks*. Nobody knows why we experience them after birth, but rest assured, they don't last forever! Usually just the first few months after birth.

> The itchy legs I had for several months after I gave birth. I did not have an explanation, but lo and behold, itchy ass legs every night. Eventually it just went away.
>
> —Leah

Not only is postpartum itching normal, but postpartum hives can be as well, even if you aren't someone who typically has sensitive skin. The itching or hives can be from any plethora of things, but the most common are changes in hormone levels, poor diet, weakened immune system, or hypersensitivity to allergens (thanks to pregnancy). Don't worry; hives and itching disappear as quickly as they appear, and usually without any treatment, although I would recommend having some Benadryl on hand!

# CHAPTER 8

# THE MOM DIAPER

You are probably asking yourself a question along these lines right now: *Why on God's green earth is there a chapter called "The Mom Diaper"? There is no way I am wearing a diaper, and why would I need to?*

That was what I thought when I first had a child and people recommended that I buy Depends, which are essentially adult diapers. *Why would I need to buy Depends?* I wondered. *Am I going to lose bladder control?* Let me preface this portion by saying that it is mostly for ladies who have vaginal deliveries.

When you vaginally deliver a baby, you bleed (often quite a lot), and you may or may not have an episiotomy. After you deliver, the nursing staff will give you what they might affectionately refer to as "Victoria Secret panties." In reality, these are mesh boy-short looking things designed for holding the world's largest pad. This pad will make you feel like you have a pillow between your legs, and it will shift every time you so much as *think* about moving. You will wake up with blood in the bed, your pad stuck to your leg, and a god-awful wedgie thanks to those mesh "panties." It is in that moment that you will realize why people recommend Depends.

> Wear Depends! They are so much better than nylon one-size-fits-all panties and the chunky, ever-moving pads the hospital gives you.
>
> —Heather

Depends are a discreet adult diaper made for people with incontinence issues, but they are also all the rage with new moms. You can slip on a pair of underwear-looking Depends and rest easy knowing that everything will stay where it belongs while you toss and turn trying to sleep. When you wear them out of the house, you will not feel like you have a pillow shoved between your legs, and will not have to worry about looking down and seeing your pad coming out of the bottom of your pants. Best of all, every evening you can just toss them in the trash!

> I determined after my fourth child that I did not use more than one package of Depends. Nobody told me how long you need to wear them after giving birth.
>
> —Elizabeth

This goes back to my earlier statement, which is that every woman is different, so postpartum looks different for each of us. I was given one package of adult diapers (can we call it a less embarrassing word, like garment . . . yes, I will refer to adult diapers as garments for the rest of this paragraph!) and didn't even use the whole package—I think it had like twenty in it—but some women may need one to two garments a day for up to six weeks. My recommendation would be to start with just one pack. If you need more, you can get more when your first pack runs low, but you aren't stuck with twenty packs of "garments" if you end up only needing one.

> Pads straight from the refrigerator feel wonderful as a pantyliner up against episiotomy stitches.
> —Stephanie

I discussed this in an earlier chapter but yes, all of the "yes" to this comment! I put my pads in the freezer instead of using an ice pack, which can be bulky, uncomfortable, and even painful with its sharp edges. Pads are a made-to-fit ice pack. They lay nicely in your underwear and even have a sticky strip to keep them in place. The frozen pad really helps with any burning or pain from stitches.

# CHAPTER 9

# BRINGING BABY HOME

For me, bringing my brand-new baby home was stressful, whether it was my first baby or my fifth. I didn't want to leave the comfort of the hospital where help was just a click away; my mind would conjure up everything that could go wrong, and I wished I could bring my doctor and team of nurses home with me. Yet as worried as I was, I was also excited to get home and start my life with my new addition, not to mention being able to sleep without being woken up every two hours by a doctor or nurse. My biggest fear with all my children was that first drive home. They were so tiny and innocent, and I felt like they were not protected in that big car seat. I sat in the back fretting over my husband's abilities to transport us home safely. Then once we got home, I stressed about my ability to adequately take care of my sweet, helpless baby.

My babies all slept the entire time we were in the hospital. I didn't think I would experience lack of sleep or backward sleep schedules. Then as soon as we got home it was like a switch turned on, and they suddenly decided to be up all night. I always joke that my kids just took over the role of keeping me up at night since I no longer had the nurses to do it! As soon as you bring baby home, you have to start sleep-training your baby to sleep at night and not during the day. You must remember that while in the womb your movements during the day rocked baby to sleep, which meant your baby was up during the night while you slept. Therefore, when your baby is born, it is trained to sleep during the day and stay awake at night, something that you need to work on in order to flip-flop.

> You can buy those head rests for your baby at any [baby] store or on Amazon. There are some that have three rolls, so they grow with your baby. It helps eliminate the head flopping.
>
> —Lori

I highly recommend you purchase a head support liner for the inside of your car seat, so you do not have to freak out when you see your baby's head flop to the side while you're on the road. I will tell you a funny little story about the first time this happened with my first son. I didn't know that they had neck supports, so I obviously didn't have one. One day, my husband was getting our son out of the car and I heard him say, "Oh my gosh." I looked back and there he was, cradling my sons head in his hands. I screamed and rushed over because I thought his head had fallen off (the rest of his body was covered by a blanket, don't judge). My husband looked at me like I had two heads and said, "What? His head was flopped over to the side."

> Buy a mirror so you can see your rear-facing baby while you are driving. They make some specifically for that reason.
>
> —Juli

I loved having a mirror for my kids. I would angle it so that I could see the mirror from my rearview mirror. Then I could look up and check on my baby every few seconds—I mean minutes—without needing to turn around.

> When you first come home, have someone limit the time that visitors can stay. You will be so exhausted.
>
> —Janice

This further comment comes from my friend Bethany, who said, "If your friends and family are anything like mine, when you get home, you will have an entire welcoming committee . . . a welcoming committee that does not seem to leave for the first two weeks. All I wanted to do was take a shower, sleep, and be with my new baby. Instead, I felt like a party host. It is absolutely okay to limit visitors and even ask for no visitors at all. Sure, somebody may get their feelings hurt, but you will maintain your sanity and that is all that matters."

I agree with Bethany; it is important to set boundaries for you and your new baby. I will add a caveat to that though: if people want to come visit you and your new baby, utilize those

You Forgot to Mention

moments. Have them hold your baby so you can take a shower, get something to eat, or even run to the grocery store. By doing this, you both win: they get to see and hold your new baby, and you can get some things done or just take a moment to breathe. You can also schedule times, like not allowing people at the house between the hours of six in the evening and ten in the morning, or only allowing people to come over during a certain timeframe. This gives your family those one-on-one bonding moments while also allowing others to be part of those first few days.

> You can say no to people visiting. Get used to feeling like everything you do is wrong.
>
> —Katie

With me, I enjoyed having people come over because my husband worked when I had my boys and when I had my daughter, I was a single parent. I had no problem inviting someone over then using that time to take a nap while they loved on my baby. When my first son was a baby, my mom would come over during her lunch hour so I could nap or shower while she rocked her new grandson. Then she would slip him into his swing and sneak out when it was time for her to go. She may not have realized how beneficial that was to me, but it was truly the difference between keeping and losing my sanity.

# CHAPTER 10

# WHY DO I FEEL THIS WAY?

Postpartum depression was something I experienced with both my first child and my last (but not in between). After the birth of my first child, I could not understand why I was experiencing such extreme mood swings. I ricocheted between uncontrollable crying, anger, and insomnia. I was so happy to have my sweet baby with me at last, yet I also felt down all the time, and often all I wanted to do was cry. I did not realize at the time that I was experiencing postpartum depression (or PPD), something that eighty percent of new moms experience. If so many people (that's right, ten percent of partners get PPD as well) are experiencing some form of PPD, why is it not more widely talked about?

While some women are told to expect the wild hormone ride that leads up to birth, it's less common to talk about the impact these hormones have on us when they begin to drop after birth and how it can affect our daily lives. New parents need to be educated on the various levels of PPD and when to seek treatment. In my opinion, *baby blues* is a quaint way of describing the mood swings almost all new moms may feel in the days immediately following the birth of a child. These moods may range from sadness and feeling overwhelmed to general crankiness, but they usually go away after a week or two without any intervention from a doctor. If you expect to get baby blues, if or when you begin to feel those fluctuations in hormones you will be prepared. However, if you don't know to expect them then that lack of understanding just adds to your already sensitive state.

Postpartum depression is more serious, lasts much longer, and often requires the intervention of a doctor. Symptoms of PPD can range anywhere from extreme mood swings to feelings of hopelessness and bonding issues. Just like depression, PPD often needs to be treated through medication or counseling. If you think you may be struggling with PPD, or if you struggle with thoughts of hurting yourself or your baby, contact your ob-gyn right away. There are medications you can take and other psychological treatments, including counseling, that you can undergo that will help you while your body and mind cope with this new life. You may find that after a few weeks, you no longer need those interventions. Or maybe you will realize you like yourself better on medication or in counseling, or both. Either way, there is no reason you have to suffer alone.

No one mentioned the hormone changes you go through *after* having a baby.

—Amanda

Many years and a couple of babies later, after the birth of my final baby, a little girl, I began to experience the disordered mood symptoms I had after the birth my first child—only this time, they were even worse. By then I had been in the medical field for ten years and had spent three of them working in gynecology.

So, when I began to recognize those negative feelings and realized that I was experiencing roller coaster mood swings, I knew what I was dealing with. And thank goodness I did, because this time the feelings did not go away on their own, and eventually my doctor had to prescribe me something. I do not feel like I am weaker for needing help; instead, I feel emboldened. I recognized that something was wrong and sought treatment instead of trying to cover up my feelings, which was something I had always done in the past.

Doctors are not quite sure what triggers PPD: whether it is due to the sudden change in hormones, a genetic disposition, or even an issue with a woman's thyroid after birth. The good news is that just because you had it with one pregnancy does not mean it will happen every time. I believe I developed PPD with my first son because of the complications I experienced during the birthing process. Whereas with my final child, my only daughter, I believe my PPD was due to the sudden absence of extra estrogen in my body after nine months of carrying around a tiny estrogen pump.

One thing I can tell you for sure, though, is that whether you are naturally inclined to experience bouts of depression, extenuating circumstances bring on PPD, or whatever the case may be, it is *always* okay to seek support or treatment. Some of the best support you will get is your significant other because oftentimes they will feel something similar to what you are feeling. Like many things that take place in our bodies during and after pregnancy, you cannot decide if you will or will not get PPD (or baby blues). You can put in your birthing plan under the list of things you do not want to happen, but it will remain unfortunately beyond your control. However, you *are* able to address it if it occurs.

> No one told me forty weeks of hormone buildup reverts back in less than forty-eight hours.
>
> —Kate

You have to appreciate the extreme changes a woman goes through during pregnancy, birth, and postpartum. Consider how that process affects every person differently. During pregnancy, hormone levels peak just to plummet after giving birth. These fluctuations in hormones are not easy to deal with: imagine experiencing PMS (premenstrual syndrome), but for nine months! Your oxytocin levels spike as baby is coming out, then level off again once baby is born, and this experience is a hormonal and emotional roller coaster not to be underestimated. Later, as your body is adjusting to post-pregnancy hormones, it must also adjust to sleep deprivation and even more overwhelming emotions.

Or perhaps you do not have postpartum depression, you just feel disconnected; you do not want to take medications, but you are struggling with bonding, feelings of depression, or other minor symptoms. It's still a good idea to consult with your doctor or healthcare professional, but there are other options as well. We live in the technology era, and Facebook does not disappoint! There are online support groups and chat rooms for every type of mama (and daddy) out there, and you just might find that you are not the only struggling with those particular feelings. However, as we all know, there are plenty of well-intentioned people and plenty of good advice on the Internet . . . but there is also plenty of the opposite. Please take anything you come across online with common sense, caution, a grain of salt, and the assurance there are professionals who can confirm or disprove anything that feels "wrong."

> Sometimes postpartum depression does not present as "depression." Sometimes it presents as anxiety, like rearranging your whole living situation so you never have to go up and down your stairs because you are afraid you will drop the baby.
>
> —Julie

> When you feel like crying, try laughing instead.
> —Olive

Okay, a bit confusing right? I just spent an entire chapter telling you to embrace your struggles and now you are reading instructions to just laugh it off. Laughing things off sometimes doesn't work—let's face it, in the end stages of pregnancy or the beginning stages of mommy hood, it mostly doesn't work. However, there are times when laughing is the best medicine.

You may not laugh immediately, but always keep the thought *this could be a memory* in the back of your head. Something may make you want to scream, but years down the road it will be a funny story your kids love to hear over and over.

# CHAPTER 11

# BONDING

There I was, laying in my hospital bed, holding the most beautiful little baby in the world. He had ten perfect little fingers, ten perfect little toes, and the blondest shock of hair standing straight up on his head. As I lay there, caressing his little cheek, I felt . . . nothing. It was like I was holding a stranger's child, not the baby I had carried in my womb for the last nine months. Even worse, he seemed to feel the same way. He cried when I touched him and would rather die than nurse from my bosom. I could not understand why my heart was not melting completely like it had with my first child—I should have been over the moon!

How many people had told me I would "forget the pain the moment the baby was born," or that my world "would change the moment they came into my life"? I was supposed to spend my days lying around, soaking in the presence of this perfect little human I had created while feeling a little pitter-patter in my heart. Instead, I did not want to be around him. He cried incessantly, and I just knew this newborn baby hated me. I did not understand how he could be so different to his older brother, a child who was born less than two years before him.

109

At the time, I didn't tell anybody about my bonding issues with my son. I was so embarrassed and ashamed that I could not bond with him, and I worried that people would think less of me if they ever found out. I wondered constantly what was wrong with me and wished there was some magical way to make me feel something, *anything* for this sweet boy. I suffered in silence for years. Every time I looked at my son, my heart ached. As he got older, it was obvious that our relationship was vastly different from that of his brother and I. Kenny loved cuddling and even slept with me for years, whereas Andy recoiled when I would touch him.

I wish that I had been able to tell somebody back then what I was going through. I would have discovered that I was not alone, and that one third of new moms experience bonding issues. I spent the next eight years intentionally destroying my relationship with a good guy, just because of his desire to have kids and my fear that I wouldn't bond with said baby. All of this stress could have been avoided had I known that bonding issues were normal and could be fixed.

It was not until I wrote my first book that I admitted I had bonding issues with my son. I remember bawling my eyes out as I wrote about it, overcome with this guilt that had accompanied me for the last twelve years of his life. When I was researching this book, I began to hear about the experiences of other parents that were also or had also experienced bonding issues. I was shocked to find out that I was not the only mom who struggled with bonding. I was even able to connect with other parents and learn what they had done and were doing to bond with their children.

I got pregnant with Andrew in an attempt to save a failing marriage. Giving birth didn't help, and the issues we experienced with our new baby just added to the issues we were having. Another contributor (one I wouldn't learn for twelve years) was the fact that Andrew is a genius and has ADHD. His inability to connect with people goes far beyond me: it is hard-wired into him. I had no way of knowing these things when he was a baby, but now that we know that this is just who he is, I am better able to address it. I have learned to show my son love in ways that don't include big hugs and cuddling. On the other hand, I have also learned to appreciate his way of showing affection which, of course, does not include touch.

> I had trouble bonding with my first child because my labor and delivery were so hard and were such a traumatic experience for me. I needed time to "forgive him" for everything I went through. I understand it was not his fault, and he did not do it intentionally, but it is important to acknowledge how we feel . . . and not pretend we are okay when we are not. I tried to bury my feelings at first, but once I acknowledged those feelings, I could deal with them and begin the healing process. It all happened within the first days of giving birth, and those days are a complete whirlwind, as any new mom can attest to. My son is twelve now. He is my best bud, and I adore him.
>
> **—Ashley**

Throughout my pregnancy with my daughter, I feared that she and I would not bond. I even planned on only taking off work the weekend she was born because I was certain I would feel nothing for my baby. I was bringing a baby into the world as a single mom, and there were so many outside factors bearing down on me during my pregnancy that I was certain I would not have the mental capacity to love a baby. Of course, because I feared about my inability to bond, I also worried that if I did not bond with her, who would? I spent my entire pregnancy racked with anxiety that the same thing would happen with her that had happened with my son all those years ago.

The dreaded day came when I went into labor: there I was, alone in a hospital room, ready to give birth to my baby. I have a video someone took at the hospital right after I gave birth to my daughter. In the video, the nurses lay my baby girl in my arms for the first time, and immediately I break down sobbing. Of course, when someone else watches the video, they think I am crying tears of joy. In reality, I was crying tears of relief, tears of guilt, and tears of all these other emotions that flooded out of my body after nine months of worrying. The second they put her in my arms, I felt like my heart had exploded out of my chest, just as all my pregnancy books had promised I was "supposed" to feel.

I was and still so am grateful that I didn't have issues bonding with my daughter. However, that experience added to my guilt over my bonding issues with my son. I never wanted my son to think he was anything outside of amazing, or that he had done anything to not deserve the same reaction his siblings got. What I have learned is that each child and each relationship is different. My bonding issue was a combination of outside factors and my son's reaction to my touch. When I learned to appreciate that our relationship was different, I was able to bond with my son.

What all this has taught me, and what I want readers to take away from this story, is that bonding issues are normal. It is okay to have them, and there are ways to maneuver and even mend those issues. What isn't okay is burying those feelings and thinking they will just go away, because they won't. Guilt, anger, or any extreme emotion does not magically go away; it just may morph into something else. The best thing you can do is find support either in peers, with loved ones, or even a counselor—anyone or any platform where you are going to feel safe enough to be open and honest and address those feelings.

> I experienced bonding issues with my first child. To this day, I still cannot seem to bond with him, and I do not know why. I hate myself for it and try everything to fix the issues, but it is so bad for me that I cannot even stand being hugged by him. He is so sweet and loving, but sometimes I have to just tell him that I can't be touched because I don't want him to know I can't stand his touch. I do not have this issue with my other two and I do not understand why it is this way with him.
>
> —Krista

I understand how hard this quote can be and how it can make people fear that this will be them as well. However, it doesn't have to be. Support, communication, and professional help can get you through this severe bonding issue and help you determine the true issue at play.

I had no bond with my first child. I cried myself to sleep every night and tried to blame my feelings on my PPD. I didn't try to hide it. Instead I would talk to my husband about it, and he would help me get through those moments. Communicating those feelings to others and accepting any advice they may have really helps any parent dealing with bonding issues. It took me five months to actually realize that I had a child. I have never liked taking care of other people, and he was no exception. However, he has changed that for me over the years. He has taught me how to love others and how to care for others. The bonding issue was all me, and that amazing little boy helped me through.

—Nay

I want to add a caveat to this comment: not every woman is bred with this great desire to be a mom, and many women choose not to have kids because they lack this desire. Whether a woman wants to have kids or not is completely her prerogative, and she should never be forced to do something she doesn't feel an innate desire to do. I have met many women who did not want kids, ultimately got guilted into having one, and then regretted it. Those scenarios are not fair to the woman, her significant other, or the child. In this case, Nay was able to learn and grow from the experience of being "forced" into caregiving, but I don't want to give the illusion that this will happen for everyone.

> I experienced bonding issues with my daughter for the first few months. At the time, I could not understand why I could possibly be having issues bonding with my baby. Later on, I realized I was unknowingly blaming my PPD on her. Once I sought out professional help and got on medication for my anxiety and depression, I was able to start the bonding process. Now our relationship could not be any stronger; she is my everything.
>
> —Chloe

I will add here a note that, if you haven't already, you should take the time to really read and process the information in this book regarding postpartum depression. PPD can manifest itself in so many ways, including anger, resentment, and hostility. One can never assume to know what feelings will manifest, who those feelings will be aimed at, or why. However, if you have prepared yourself for the possibility that you will get baby blues or PPD, you can address those emotions sooner and will be less likely to feel like there is something wrong with you, your baby, or your ability to bond.

I still feel like I am looking out for someone else's baby at times. He is two months old, and I love him to pieces, but I get so irritated when he wants attention and all his basic needs have been met already. I am not a clingy person and do not really like being touched all that much, so it is difficult for me to hold him knowing he does not actually need anything but is just looking for some love and connection. I blame myself for it. He deserves love and affection in abundance; I just can't give it to him.

—Ulyssa

Feelings like these are far more common than people realize; they just aren't spoken about as frequently. We have all heard the term "maternal instincts," the term that covers the innate response women are supposed to have to children and the reason moms seem to have "eyes on the back of their heads." For some women, those maternal instincts kick in years before having kids; for others, they don't kick in until after the baby is born. But what happens when they don't kick in at all?

During my career in the fire service, fellow firefighters would always joke that they needed to clone me or would ask why there weren't more women around like me. In their mind, I was a good-looking (their opinions, definitely not mine!) female without all the drama. They saw a woman who chose drinks with the guys over manicures, and my general lack of empathy and emotions was perfect for the fire house. However, what they did not see was my inability to connect with my sons in a way that moms should or the way that I so wanted to but just couldn't. The firefighters couldn't see my inability to maintain relationships or create bonds with other women. And, yeah, maybe sometimes a wife's emotions can be a bit "annoying" or whatever you want to call it, but what is more annoying is a woman who cannot emotionally connect with you. My personality may have been great for the fire house, but it sucked at home.

My ability to be "one of the guys" and my inability to coddle and show empathy to others was due to a chemical imbalance happening inside my body. I had always had low estrogen levels, and each time I became pregnant with a boy, my estrogen levels got lower and lower. I was like interacting with a brick wall. I was just like the mom in this quote: I was physically revolted by people's need for love and attention outside of their basic needs.

I did not write this book with the intentions of it being one of my stuffy medical textbooks from college, but in the same sense, I also know knowledge is power, and people feel far more in control when they know what's happening inside them. So on that note, let's talk about why I was the way I was, and maybe why you are that way too. Estrogen is this amazing group of sex hormones that does everything from helping you get pregnant, to breast growth (don't mind if I do!), and everything in between ... including regulating your mood.[1] Estrogen affects your mood by its very close relationship to serotonin, the "mood-balancing" chemical. Estrogen promotes the production of serotonin, so when your estrogen is low, so is your serotonin.[2] That's when things start to go bad. Women with low estrogen levels experience depression, lack emotional connections, and have severe anger outbursts (that was the worst for me).

I got lucky because I ended up getting pregnant with a girl, and my body began producing estrogen again, but this isn't the case with all women. As luck would have it though, we now have the options of estrogen therapy and receiving estrogen. However, some women choose not to do that and choose to learn how to live with their low estrogen, and that is perfectly fine too. Women who lack empathy or maternal instincts can still be great parents, they just need to work a little harder at the emotional attachment. For Ulyssa, that means understanding the importance of holding a baby and knowing the benefits of holding babies despite all their physical needs being met. For me, my lack of empathy meant that I needed mentors in my life who could speak into situations and help me respond correctly. I cannot say that the addition of estrogen has completely fixed my inability to coddle, but it has made me less emotionless.

The biggest contributor has been my husband, a man who had already started raising daughters when we met. He is now my mentor: when our daughter gets a "boo-boo" (not something I believe is worth crying over) he will literally sit her in my lap and wrap my arms around her, whereas I would typically pat her on the head, tell her she's okay, and send her away. A colleague and dear friend of mine also struggles with empathy issues; for her, counseling is what works best. Her lack of empathy and dislike of being touched affects her relationship with both her spouse and her children, so she uses a counselor as her mentor. The counselor helps her learn to mentally control her revulsion to physical touch, and address the issues that are causing it.

If you are one of the many people that battle with these feelings, understand that you are not alone and there are people that can help you cope with being a new parent.

I could not bond with my second child for almost two months. I resented her, almost, because I had to have a C-section with her. They had to put me asleep, so I missed the entire birth, and when I woke up, I felt like they handed me someone else's child. In the hospital, I could not do anything on my own and was in extreme amounts of pain. I could not do basic things like pick her up or put her down. When someone would hand her to me for feedings, I physically could not put her down afterwards. I had to ask for help on everything—and as someone who does everything on my own and hates asking for help, it did something to me. My partner would not help me (and was acting like a jerk because I was asking for help) which meant I began resenting both him *and* her. I did not start liking her until I began feeling better and started being able to do things on my own again. I feel really bad about it still.

—Rose

I had such a hard time bonding with my first. Finally, I realized that breastfeeding was putting a barrier between us, since I was forcing myself to do it but hated it. Once I stopped breastfeeding, I became a better mom and was able to bond with her. She is my bestie now! You *have* to do what works for you and your baby, not what others think you should do.

—Brittany

I struggled to bond with my second child due to really bad PPD that lingered for years. I am so much better now, and my life revolves around my daughter. I am not sure what caused the severe PPD—if it was the fact that I had another child and was feeling overwhelmed, or if it was a chemical imbalance. Whatever it was, I am glad we were able to work through it. She is the sweetest, most gentle human being ever, and I am so glad to say that now she and I are closer than most parents are with their children.

—Hunter

It seemed like my daughter wanted nothing to do with me for the first three years of her life, and that made it so hard to bond with her. She basically only cried when I was around and would immediately stop as soon as her dad came around. It went on like that for the first two or so years, but now we are best friends, and she is a total mama's girl. She always wants to be around me— but there are still days where she just wants her daddy and that is okay. Especially when it is the middle of the night and I want to sleep!

—Laura

I am going to let you in on a little secret that someone told me before I had children, which ultimately saved me a lot of heartache with my kids (especially my daughter). A young lady was complaining that she was a stay-at-home mom, did everything for her new baby, and her baby's first word was "Dada." This wise woman chuckled and said, "I didn't mind my kid saying 'Dada' as their first word. It meant in the middle of the night when they were up crying and screaming 'Dada,' I could elbow him and say, 'The baby is calling you,' and roll over and fall back asleep." The wise woman told the young girl to take it as a blessing and use those moments as a chance to do something for herself, rather than take it as a personal offense.

My daughter was—and is—a daddy's girl. She will walk right past me to go ask him to do something for her. She adores the ground he walks on, and there are still so many opportunities where jealousy gets the better of me. Then I stop and remember the wise woman's words. So instead of being jealous, I try to appreciate their bonds and think of the positives, like "at least I don't have to carry her all the time." It may sound stupid, but it makes me feel better. My daughter is my best friend in the whole world now and I love every second I get with her, but she still prefers her dad most of the time—and that is okay! What makes her happy makes me happy.

I bonded with my first immediately, but am only now bonding with my second, who is six months old. It is hard, no doubt. I was never angry or regretful for my second child; quite the opposite, I am thrilled he is here! Bonding issues just happen sometimes. I have terrible PPD and am getting help to address my PPD. The more I address my issues, the easier bonding is getting.

—Cindy

> I could not bond with my first child at the beginning. It was like having a very whiney roommate that I had to take care of. The birth was traumatic, so even holding him in the hospital I did not feel a connection. I finally admitted my feelings to my husband, and shockingly enough he told me he felt the same way! I felt less alone when I learned that, and we were able to talk it through. We were even able to make jokes to lighten the mood when we were both feeling that way. Around month two, my son smiled for the first time, and it was like something just clicked for both me and my husband. We both fell in love with that little boy, like everything we had gone through had been worth it, just to see him smile.
>
> **—Stephanie**

Thank you to all the moms (and dads) who were willing to be honest about their bonding issues. I know it is hard to admit that you were not just head over heels in love with your child from the moment they were born like you are "supposed" to be, but if we all listened to what we were "supposed" to be doing, we'd miss out on a lot of things only we can experience and only we can offer. I think it takes a lot of love and courage to admit when things are not all ribbons and roses, and even more courage to get help.

As I and so many others in this chapter have said, attachment issues can come from a myriad of different sources, can manifest themselves is various ways, last anywhere from days to years, and can be treated or solved through a plethora of different avenues.[3] Whether bonding issues stem from a traumatic birth, or a either a parent or child lacks the capacity to love in a "conventional" manner, there are ways to cope with this season of life. There are professionals who are trained to help parents (and children) through these difficulties. In fact, 33 percent of new parents experience bonding issues when asked, and one in ten new mothers said they were embarrassed to admit it or seek professional help for their inability to bond.[4] This means that there are so many people out there that are either also going through their own battle or can offer advice and support.

# CHAPTER 12

# THE JOY OF BREASTS

Normally I like to open each chapter with a funny story, but I want to open this one with a little information. We have all heard the old adage "breast is best," but I much prefer the one becoming more popular in the millennial generation: "fed is best." In this chapter, we will discuss the pros and cons of breastfeeding, but we will also go over what to do if you cannot or chose not to breastfeed. Yes, breastfeeding is a magical experience and such a great time to bond with your baby, and breastmilk has some irreplaceable properties, but not everyone has the desire or ability to nurse, and that is okay. In this chapter, I will tell some personal stories about my issues with breastfeeding and the scenario that changed my mind from "breast is best" to "fed is best." My goal is not to change your mind; my goal is to educate you so that you go into motherhood feeling confident and prepared.

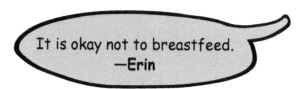

It is okay not to breastfeed.
—Erin

Breastfeeding (if you so choose) is not beautiful and cute like on TV. It is messy. It takes practice and struggles and sometimes tears and formula and that is okay. (I did not get it right until baby number three.)

—Melissa

If you choose to breastfeed, it is exhausting. Everyone has their opinion on it, but I was never told how dang hard and tiring it was. Especially on the days that all they wanted to do was eat.

—Jessica

Breastfeeding was the single most stressful thing in the beginning. Everyone said it would get better for us, but it just did not. I ended up exclusively pumping because she just would not stay latched and would freak out every time I tried to nurse.

—Anna

The first time I nursed my first son, it was the most magical moment I had ever experienced. He latched so perfectly, and I loved looking down seeing my sweet new baby suckling. The moment of sheer bliss lasted about five seconds, until the contractions started. Yes, *contractions*. It was like being in labor all over again, yet this time my baby was in my arms! As we discussed in chapter 6, I later learned that those contractions were my uterus contracting back to its normal size, and that breastfeeding stimulated those contractions . . . I just wasn't aware of this until I experienced it. Feeling contractions during breastfeeding can last up to several weeks after your baby is born. However, the intensity of those contractions will decrease as time goes on.

> Contractions during nursing got worse with each kid! By baby number three, I thought I was going to die every time I nursed for the first forty-eight hours or so.
>
> **—Suzie**

> First time I breastfed, it felt like someone or something was reaching into my body from the breast to my spine and pulling my spine out through my breasts. It was the weirdest feeling.
>
> **—Autumn**

In the hospital before giving birth, a nurse will typically ask you if you are planning to breastfeed. They ask this so that once your baby is born, they can immediately begin assisting you with feeding. I have learned throughout the years (and multiple babies) that they will try to get you to attempt breastfeeding whether you planned to or not. This whole process can be a bit intimidating and extremely overwhelming, especially if you are modest or prefer complete strangers not to see your breasts.

Someone will come and inform you that it is feeding time, and before you know what is happening, they are man-handling your breast and popping it into your baby's mouth.

This person is the lactation nurse, and their sole responsibility is to ensure your baby is latching correctly. The lactation nurse makes sure that your baby receives the vital nutrients they need within that first hour of life, and that the mom doesn't give up on breastfeeding before giving it a real chance because she feels like she isn't doing it correctly. It isn't widely taught to new moms how important it is to get baby fed within the first hour, or how mind-blowingly beneficial colostrum is (don't worry, I will explain what that is shortly), so it may seem a bit invasive to have someone "all up in your face" right after a tiring birthing experience. Lactation nurses understand the significance of this first hour, and they truly have both mom's and baby's best interests in mind.

Trust me when I say, completely outside of the benefits for my baby, I would rather someone man-handle my breasts and ensure my baby is latching correctly than go through the pain I experienced when my children didn't latch correctly. Eventually you learn a certain pain is specific to latching issues and can adjust accordingly, but when nursing is new to you, you may not realize that is what is happening. Your lactation nurse is there to ensure that you don't have to experience that pain full time until you throw in the towel. Just so that we are all on the same page, latching is when the baby's mouth is on the full lower portion of the nipple's areola in the appropriate way.

If a baby is not latching—they are just getting a small portion of the nipple, the wrong spot on the nipple, or even the wrong spot on the breast altogether—it can create frustration for both mom and baby, as well as significant pain for the mom. More so than the pain and frustration that latching issues can cause, they also create a chain reaction within your and your baby's bodies. When your baby nurses, it needs to be able to get enough milk to gain weight. The amount of milk the baby removes tells your body whether it needs to increase, decrease, or maintain milk production. So, if your baby isn't removing enough milk, they will not gain the weight they need to be healthy, and your milk will begin to dwindle.

Nobody told me how hard breastfeeding could actually be. As a first-time mom, I felt like such a failure because my baby could not latch. I thought everyone could do it automatically and there was something terribly wrong with me.

My second baby was a breeze when it came to nursing, and I learned that not all babies will be able to latch. There are many causes for that and none of them are because you are a bad mom.

**—Alicia**

Every newborn is different. I remember sobbing after my third child was born because I could not get them to latch. It all worked out, but not without the help of some really amazing nurses.

**—Kristie**

My daughter was born with a tongue-tie, which means that the lingual frenulum (that small piece of tissue under your tongue that connects your tongue to the bottom of your mouth) is either too close to the tip of the tongue, too short, or too tight. Because of her tongue-tie, we had to work harder at nursing, which caused my already low milk supply to drop even further. A tongue-tie is easily fixed with an outpatient procedure that is usually done within a few minutes. Normally, a baby will begin nursing adequately within twenty minutes following the procedure. My daughter's tongue-tie was not bad, but because it caused issues with nursing we chose to have the procedure. Typically if the tongue-tie is not bad, your child's pediatrician will give you the option on whether or not you want it fixed.

I wish someone had told me about lip and tongue-ties. A baby with either is going to have difficulty nursing, and you would never know this if someone did not point it out. Luckily our pediatrician noticed it right away and fixed it. She [my baby] nursed like a champ after the procedure. I was surprised to learn it was an easy outpatient procedure.

—Anna

Despite my first son adequately latching, by day three, my nipples were these bloody little stumps. They hurt even when they weren't being touched, and breastfeeding became so painful that I cried whenever it was time to breastfeed. I finally called my ob-gyn, who recommended nipple cream to help with the chafing. Although the creams helped, my nipples were still chafed and raw for the first few weeks of nursing, something that I didn't realize was perfectly normal. You can minimize the chafing and eliminate the bleeding by applying a thin layer of nipple cream every time you are finished nursing.

> They say breastfeeding is beneficial, but surely do not tell you how your nipples will feel.
>
> —Luzeria

> If you are breastfeeding and your nipples start bleeding, your baby may spit up blood . . . that was a freak out!
>
> —Robi

> Nipple chafing. Whether your baby is latching correctly or not (if you nurse), you are going to get some nipple chafing the first few days. Slap some coconut oil (or other safe salve) on there and relax. It will go away after a few days. Oh, but make sure you get some pads for in your bra because of leakage.
>
> —Joan

Your lactation nurse will also ensure that you are producing colostrum and will explain to you what it feels like when your milk drops. Colostrum is your body's "first stage" of breast milk;

it helps your baby to poop—which clears out their system from all the things they ingested invitro—and provides the necessary nutrients for your newborn baby to gain weight. As your baby grows, your milk supply will as well . . . or it should. One of the main reasons that new mothers stop breastfeeding is pain, but another one is a lack of milk production. For me personally, I was a milk-geyser with my first child: I could have nursed an entire preschool. However, with each child I produced less and less milk. By the time my daughter was born, I was fighting to produce two ounces of breast milk a day. By the time my daughter was a month old, I was supplementing, and by two months I was completely dependent on formula. This takes me back to my ongoing advice: no matter how many kids you have, each pregnancy, birth, and baby is different.

My sister-in-law (SIL) and I were pregnant with our sons at the same time. For her it was her first, and for me it was my second. A few weeks after both our sons were born, my mom, my grandma, and I made the trek out to California to meet my new nephew. When we got there and saw him, we were horrified. My son was a fat little cherub of a baby, and he starkly contrasted the skeleton that was my new nephew. My nephew was so skinny and sickly-looking compared to my son, and it was glaringly obvious to my mom, my grandma, and me that this child was grossly malnourished.

My mom asked my SIL if she was exclusively breastfeeding. Of course, she was. Further into the conversation, my SIL explained to us that her son was nursing nearly all day: she said he never slept, constantly cried, and was only content when latched onto her breast. We expressed our concerns that her son was not getting enough nutrients and needed to be supplemented. My SIL told us that her doctor had assured her that her baby would get everything he needed from her breast milk and that breastfed babies didn't need to be supplemented. What her doctor didn't explain to her is that she may never produce milk, therefore her baby would not be getting what he needed.

A quick trip to the doctor confirmed our suspicions—her milk had never dropped. Despite her continuous nursing, her baby was slowly dying from malnutrition. Once they began bottle-feeding my nephew, he began to gain weight, stopped crying incessantly, and began sleeping longer between feedings. I honestly cannot say why her pediatrician didn't catch what was going on, nor does it matter. What matters is that my nephew is now a happy and healthy thirteen-year-old because his mom chose to listen when someone voiced their concern, and knew that a fed baby is more important than where the milk is coming from.

Do not give up on breastfeeding, and if need be, see a lactation specialist. It will take a little while for your milk to come in, and that is okay. The baby's stomach is ridiculously small, and in the first few days they are filling up on your colostrum.
—Emily

They failed to mention that breastfeeding produces truly little fluid in the beginning. I expected the tap to open like a spigot.
—Valerie

Minus the pain you feel as your nipples become accustomed to nursing, breastfeeding should not be painful. I was a few weeks into a horrific yeast infection on my breasts before I learned that it was not normal to be in excruciating pain every time you nurse! I was not even aware at the time that you could get a yeast infection anywhere except "down there." I also didn't know that *thrush* is another name for a yeast infection. When your baby has thrush, they can spread it to you, plus you can turn around and spread it to your significant other. Until everyone in the house is treated, your family can swap the virus around for months, making everyone in the home miserable.

My ob-gyn asked me how nursing was going during my six-week visit, and I told her I thought my son was having issues latching because every time he nursed, the pain was so intense I cried. She asked me to show her how he latched, and after one look at my nipples she said "Oh gosh! You have thrush on your nipples." She explained the vicious circle to me, provided me with an antibiotic, and told me to make appointments for my husband and son to also be treated. After a week's worth of antibiotics for my son, my husband, and I, all was right in the nursing world yet again.

Thrush or a yeast infection are not the only ailments that a nursing mom can experience. So, I implore you that if breastfeeding becomes painful or you begin feeling pain in your breasts at all while nursing, call your ob-gyn immediately and let them know what is going on. By the time we cured all my nipple issues, I was producing so much milk that I could not keep up with the production. I was changing the pads in my nursing bra at least every hour, and I remember a time that I had to stand in a restaurant bathroom and squirt milk into the toilet just to get some relief. I learned quickly that when your breasts are so full that they become hard; once you start nursing, milk can come out so fast your baby chokes on it . . . or it squirts across the room! Be careful and make sure you are alternating breasts, otherwise baby will fall asleep fat and happy on one side, and leave you with an engorged breast on the other side.

> One day I was stuck in a meeting and could not pump. I started leaking out of my armpit. Special talent right there!
>
> —Elizabeth

> I had no idea my boobs would leak! Make sure you have pads for your boobies after you give birth if you plan to breastfeed or pump.
>
> —Kristi

> Hot water from the shower will make your boobs leak breastmilk.
> —Alyssa

The tips and comments listed below may not have their own sections but are certainly worth mentioning in a book that leans toward things people *forgot to mention.*

> Take cabbage leaves, break the veins, and place one on each breast after breastfeeding when trying to ween your baby, or if you are dealing with a breast infection. It helps with pain and swelling.
>
> **—Autumn**

Research going all the way back to the 1800s says that cabbage leaves work to relieve pain and swelling. Nobody knows why, they just know it works.[1]

> Apparently, it is perfectly normal to get aroused by breastfeeding. Super awkward.
>
> **—Anonymous**

Okay, this is indeed super awkward, and definitely not something people mention to someone expecting a baby. I mean, how do you even approach this topic? "Hey, sometimes when you nurse you will get super horny and may even choose to masturbate?" Yeah, I don't think so. Instead, people just let others figure this one out on their own. But hey, that is what this book is about, right?

I understand the huge stigma surrounding women's breasts and how current society is fighting to desexualize them and portray them for what they are: a feeding mechanism for babies. I was even reprimanded at church when my first son was born because I was sitting in the pew with my new baby's head covered by a blanket. Apparently, you only cover your baby's head when breastfeeding, so my husband was pulled into the pastor's office and told to inform me that breastfeeding in church was a huge no-no. I wasn't actually breastfeeding, just had my son all snuggled up. I probably would never nurse in church anyway. But even then, I was so offended that somebody would tell me where I could feed my baby.

So, here we are, trying to make boobs a non-sexual item while also explaining that the process of breastfeeding can be sexually arousing. However, that feeling is one thousand percent normal and happens to most women, including the ones that deny it, and here is why: Say you and your significant other are about to "get it on," so he rolls over and gently begins rolling your nipples in his fingers, causing them to become erect under his touch. Now compare that scenario to your nursing baby, who, when adequately latched, will roll the nipple between their tongue and the roof of their mouth in order to stimulate milk production. It is ridiculous to think that one of these scenarios would cause sexual stimulation and the other would not, when both cause the nipple to become stimulated and the body to produce oxytocin. Furthermore, oxytocin, the hormone responsible for orgasms, is the same hormone that's responsible for milk let-down.

> I did not know breastfeeding sometimes causes you not to have a period.
>
> —Cata

Really, this quote should say "almost always." Prolactin is the hormone that causes a woman's menstrual cycle; it is also the hormone that causes milk production. As long as you are nursing, and that prolactin is working on milk production, you are less likely to ovulate or have a period. This is where the old wives' tale comes in that says nursing moms can't get pregnant. The thought was that if you aren't ovulating, you won't get pregnant, and you won't ovulate if you nurse. Although this is mostly true, I would not use nursing as your sole source of pregnancy prevention.

# CHAPTER 13

# IT'S FEEDING TIME!

Let us talk about mealtime, shall we? We've already talked about breasts, but there's plenty more when it comes to feeding. Whether the topic is bottle-feeding, supplementing, or baby's first solid foods, these stories are bound to have you giggling. Let me start out by saying again that no two children are alike. I know I have mentioned that so many times throughout this book, but this point is particularly important to keep in mind when it comes to feeding your child.

## THE BOTTLE

Let's talk formula first, and some tips and tricks that might help keep you from pulling all your hair out. When my first son was born, he breastfed until it was time to go to solids. When we tried him on solid foods, he loved everything. When we decided to switch him from the bottle to a sippy cup, he transitioned like gold. He did not even have an issue when we stopped giving him a bottle at bedtime, around his second birthday. So imagine my shock and surprise when my second son was born and then refused to eat.

Andrew was two days old when my doctor informed me that if he did not start eating, they would have to put a feeding tube in him. He refused to latch despite the guidance and assistance of all the subject matter experts at the hospital. It seemed as though Andy would rather die than have anything to do with breastfeeding. Our introduction to the bottle was not any better, and we were beginning to lose hope. Our little bundle was dropping weight by the day and was critically close to being put on a feeding tube.

We were nearly a week in when a lady at my church recommended mixing Karo syrup in his bottle. Karo syrup is like a clear, thick, sugar substance meant for baking, but we were willing to try anything to get our baby boy to eat. Eventually we figured out the perfect Karo syrup, water, and formula ratio and our son finally started eating! This fight at mealtime became the story of his life, and we faced this same type of battle until he was old enough to be told, "Eat what is served to you or don't eat at all."

Formula will keep for up to twenty-four hours, so if you can mix it in large batches, it will save you time. I used a twenty-four-ounce bottle shaker.
—Alesha

Let's talk about this tidbit of advice so there is no confusion on how long a bottle of formula will last. An untouched, unused bottle of mixed formula powder will indeed keep for up to twenty-four hours *if* stored in the refrigerator. An untouched, unused bottle of mixed formula powder is only good for two hours if left at room temperature. If your baby has already drunk some of the bottle, but does not want the rest, it is only good for one hour. If the bottle has been heated, it cannot be stored and should be thrown out within an hour of making it. Ready-to-drink liquid formula will keep for forty-eight hours once it is opened. Do not freeze formula. As always, follow your pediatrician's or the company's guidelines if you have any concerns. The formula should have instructions on the packaging.

> If using formula, the Baby Brezza is amazing!
> —Annie

The Baby Brezza is the name brand of a formula maker that automatically mixes, heats, and dispenses baby formula. Most of these machines are fairly pricey and not for people on a tight budget (although they do offer payment plans), but it is definitely something worth putting on the baby registry. Seriously, who doesn't want to push a button and have a perfectly blended bottle at their fingertips?

> Use the Kiinde bags if you are pumping. You pump, freeze, warm, and feed with same bag. Only wash the nipples.
>
> —Karla

> Do not be afraid to ask for the hospital pump, regardless of your plan to breastfeed. It can help get the milk started. Preemies do not latch well, regardless of birth weight. Mine was almost ten pounds, four weeks early. Could not latch for anything. So glad I started pumping so I could feed him that way.
>
> —Christina

Pumping . . . oh, pumping. I wish I had started pumping sooner with my daughter. A wonderful, well-kept secret that all moms need to know is that your insurance company will send you a free pump. Don't have insurance? Most state programs (like WIC) also assist in providing pumps. If all else fails, it doesn't take much digging to find a company more than willing to ship you a nice pump free of charge. For me, I knew I would end up pumping because I went back to work a week after I had my daughter, so of course my options were to stop breastfeeding or start pumping.

However, that first week that my daughter was born, she slept way more and ate way less than she should have. Side note, my daughter sleeps when she's in pain, and despite the guarantee that tongue-tie clips don't hurt, my daughter slept for two days straight after hers. So, there were so many opportunities where I should have taken advantage of the beautiful pump that my insurance company had sent me, but I didn't. I would easily go six hours without feeding Layla or pumping, which told my body I didn't need to be producing much milk. By the time I started pumping, my milk was already on its way out and I didn't have the chance to nurse/pump for long.

Christina was absolutely correct when she said to get the pump whether you think you need it or not. There are more times than not where the pump will come in handy.

## STARTING ON SOLIDS

I think one of the best parts of being a parent is watching your children experience new things. So of course, watching your child taste certain foods for the first time can be an exciting and funny experience for everyone involved. I can think of some instances in my own children's lives where I definitely should have had a camera, so here is my piece of advice in this modern technological era: always have your camera going when introducing your baby to a new food. My favorite has always been letting my babies try a lemon or lime and watching their reactions as the sour liquid hits their sensitive tastebuds.

However, as much fun as it is to experience first foods with your baby, make sure that you are doing it based on your pediatricians' guidelines. There is no set-in-stone age when children are considered "old enough" to have solids; instead, their pediatrician will focus more on signs that tell you your child is ready to try solids. Some of the things you want to look for to determine if your baby is ready for solids is if they can sit up either with some help or fully on their own but also have good head control. Of course, you can prop a newborn up and say they are sitting with assistance, but they do not have good head control. Another great indication is if your baby seems interested in what you are eating, reaches for your food, or likes to put things in their mouth. But to reiterate, ensure that your pediatrician has given you the green light before taking your baby on this new food adventure.

Once you have been given the green light to start on solids, it is always a good idea to start on simpler food like baby cereal and single ingredient baby food. I can tell you that I fed my sons jars of baby food and hand blended fresh fruits and veggies for my daughter, and no child turned out better than any other. So I truly believe that whether you decide to buy the canned baby food or make it yourself it is just a matter of preference. Another great thing to keep in mind is that your baby may not like some foods the first time they try them. It is important to keep reintroducing those foods to them—I am particularly referring to fruits and vegetables. It can take up to ten times of trying a food before your baby begins to like it.

When we began introducing solid foods to our second son, we would have to literally pry his mouth open and force feed him a bite, even if it were something we knew he liked! He is now eleven years old and although we do not have to force feed him anymore, and he is used to my "take it or leave it" mentality, he is still one of the pickiest eaters I know (second only to my daughter). You feel like such a jerk as you are sitting on your child trying to force ice cream down their throat, knowing they would like it if they would just open their mouth! However, I have learned through parenting several picky eaters that they will be only as picky as you allow them to be. Even now, I make my children try one bite of everything we cooked, even if they swear they don't like it. Oftentimes, they end up realizing they do like said food, or they like it cooked one way over another. The important thing is just to continue encouraging them to try food; as their palate matures, their tastebuds will change, and they will find foods they once hated they now like (and sometimes vice versa).

> When my son is done eating, if he has any food left on his highchair, he throws it if I do not remove it quickly enough. He gets mad because he is full and does not want it there.
>
> —Teresa

> Our first solid food go-to was baby cereal because you can water it down with breast milk, water, juice, or formula. Apples and bananas were always a hit with my kiddos, and bread-like foods were easier for them to eat with little to no teeth.
>
> —Stacey

> My nephew is almost three and is one of the pickiest toddlers ever. He eats "pizza" for almost every meal. In reality, he gets pizza rolls like twice a week, but we have to tell him that everything he's eating is pizza, or he won't eat it.
>
> —Cera

My daughter is the youngest of seven kids and we were certain that by the time she came around, we had seen it all. How wrong we were! We are used to picky eaters, so learning that she is an extremely picky eater came as no shock to us. What did come as a shock to us was her response to foods she does not like. We cannot force her to eat something she does not want (even if it is her favorite food) because she will respond by projectile vomiting all over you. Her current diet consists of ham, oranges, chocolate milk, and red skittles . . . today. Tomorrow she may throw up if we give her oranges.

> Solid foods:
> banana, avocado, and
> mashed potatoes.
> —Casey

> Both my babies did baby led weaning (where baby shares your food and learns to put bite-sized pieces in their mouth without your help), so they shared our breakfast. First solids were sharing scrambled eggs and pancakes.
> —Vannie

Baby-led weening is when you skip the step of spoon feeding and wait until the baby is old enough to grasp finger foods and bring them to their mouth. Oftentimes this includes setting the baby up in a highchair with a variation of finger foods and letting them decide which foods they want. Of course, any activity that promotes hand-eye coordination and dexterity is a win in my book.

# CHAPTER 14

# SEXY TIME

What a terribly awkward conversation, which means it is the *perfect* chapter for this book. After all, who wants to talk about their sex life (especially if they don't have one)? But I think it is important to give new parents an idea of what to expect. Unfortunately, as is the theme in this book, this is not something that people talk about unless it becomes an issue. Even then, the conversation is usually held between a doctor and their patient.

There is a reason you have a six-week check-up after having a baby: those first six weeks are hell on both your body and your hormones. Not only are your hormones all over the place, but you are physically exhausted and sore from having carried and delivered a small human. While you are enjoying the emotional intimacy of rocking, holding, and nursing your new baby, it is taking a huge toll on you both physically and hormonally. As soon as your sweet bundle of joy is outside of your body, your hormones switch from baby building to baby sustaining. This switch means that estrogen and progesterone, the hormones that spent nine months creating two of the neurotransmitters that are responsible for making a pregnant woman feel happy and calm, plummet. While those hormones are dropping like the world's fastest roller coaster, prolactin and oxytocin are in the metaphorical cart behind them, slowly creeping up the peak of the roller coaster.

As I have talked about in other chapters, prolactin is the hormone responsible for milk production. However, it also comes with some wonderful side effects that would have even the horniest of women saying "no" to sexy time. On top of the loss of libido that women feel while breastfeeding, intercourse can also be uncomfortable or even downright painful, thanks to a dry vagina. You are also getting to know your new body, which for most of us isn't an exciting time, struggling with this weird facial or body hair, and experiencing the same acne you thought you got rid of after high school.

While your body may not go back to the way it was before having children, the hair growth and acne will go away once you stop breastfeeding. However, it is understandable that a woman wouldn't feel sexy with these hormonal and body image issues in their head. This isn't just for the mom (though, yes, a woman's estrogen levels drop to crazy low levels), but men's testosterone levels drop as well. Men's testosterone levels begin dropping as soon as they get married, and continue to fall as they participate in nurturing activities.[1] I think women would feel better in those weeks after having a baby if they realized they were not the only ones struggling in the libido department.

## ADVICE FROM THE CREW

Everyone is going to feel differently after giving birth (in case I haven't said that enough times by now). I thought it would be worthwhile to share the quotes listed below in order to illustrate how much of a range there is for those of us recovering from birth while also trying to navigate our sex lives.

My sex drive is super low. I think my fear of getting pregnant again plays a huge part in that, plus finding the time and the effort it takes.

—Karla

I have a super low sex drive, but I was also a bit traumatized from the pain of a natural birth. My hormones were crazy for the first two weeks, but now at twelve weeks I am feeling a lot better, but still not in the mood.

—Meagan

Be prepared for crazy hormones. I didn't get my sex drive back until around week four. I am seven weeks postpartum now and still haven't really done anything because I am afraid of how it will feel. I have heard it can still hurt even though you get the okay from your doctor.

—Ashley

I had literally NO sex drive after my baby. At my six-week checkup I did the PPD questionnaire, and it turned out that I was suffering from PPD. After a few weeks of being on meds for that, I started to feel like my old self again, but it was still hard to fit sex in between the lack of energy, working, and working around the baby's schedule.

—Jade

The first three or so weeks, my sex drive was through the roof! I didn't even want to wait for my six-week check-up to ravage my husband. But it slowly started to go away as exhaustion and insecurities over my "new" body set in.

—Courtney

The highest sex drive I ever had was at five weeks postpartum. We were having sex twice a day for about a week.

—Taylor

My hyper sex drive is literally driving me crazy. I feel like my pre-baby self, light and energetic, and it is much easier now that I don't have a big ole belly impeding things.

—Johana

# CHAPTER 15

# I CHANGED IT LAST TIME, IT'S YOUR TURN

I think I could write an entire book solely about the adventures I had while diaper changing my four babies! When I asked other parents about the topic, the responses I received were overwhelming. I think we could all write books. Although being peed on by your baby is a rite of passage, hopefully these tips and tricks will help you limit the frequency of that christening. After three little boys, I feel like an expert in getting peed on.

## THERE HE GOES

> Little boys will pee on you. Every. Single. Time.
> —Lisa

First things first. If you do not aim "it" down when you put the diaper on a little boy, your little boy's pee will shoot right up out of the diaper. I speak from experience: it took me about two months to realize what was happening. I could not figure out why my first son's clothes would get soaked with pee, but when

I went to change his diaper, I found that it was dry. I would like to say this mishap with placement was the only time me or my husband got peed on, but alas—it was not.

> If you have a son and you are taking the diaper off, let "it" get a breath of air, and then cover it up again so he does not pee all over the place. I do not know why, but our son would always start to pee as soon as it got a breath of air.
>
> —Paul

My first son, like clockwork, would pee every single time you took his diaper off. I eventually learned to unlatch the diaper, open it, then close it again really fast. He would pee, and then we could go on with the diaper change. Of course, nearly our entire house had been "christened" before we figured that one out. The little tents they sell to put over a little boy's wee-wee? Yeah, those just shoot across the room when they pee. Save your money.

> Skip the wipe warmer. [It's a] perfect solution if you want to get peed on.
>
> —David

By the time my second and third sons came around, I was a pro. If I were changing a diaper, I would put the clean diaper under the old diaper and would toss a wet wipe over him when I took the diaper off. If he peed, the wet wipe would stop the stream from going anywhere outside the diaper, and the new diaper would catch anything the old diaper did not, saving the bed (or whatever I was changing them on).

> When changing a diaper, always put the new diaper under the old and then pull it [the old one] out. My daughter would always pee right when I took her diaper off.
>
> —Lauren

Mishaps always happen, of course, no matter how much of a pro you become. At the very least, you gain some new experience with every mishap. For instance, how many non-parents do you think have experienced the particular flavor of baby urine?

> You learn quick not to talk while a boy's thing is uncovered. That liquid does *not* taste good.[1]
>
> —Tara

> My brother was the first boy after four girls, so I learned that boys pee during diaper changes when I was nine years old. It can come out strong too— my brother watered some plants that were across the room from his changing table! They had to be at least twelve feet away!
>
> —Michelle

> Roll baby boys on their tummy when changing them. Saves on the water fountain issue.
> —Megan

Let me caveat this last quote with saying that not only have I never tried this, I would also not do it with a baby who cannot yet hold its head up as you risk your baby suffocating.

## THERE SHE GOES

Now, do not think you get off scot-free if you have a girl. Although my daughter did not shoot her pee across the room like a little boy, she loved pooping in the middle of every diaper change. And while my daughter never peed on me, her pediatrician was not as lucky. Every time we removed her diaper to check her weight, my daughter would pee, hitting her pediatrician 100 percent of the time. If I didn't know a thing or two about the brain development of infants, I would think my daughter was intentionally peeing on her pediatrician. However, I do know that newborn baby's nervous system is still maturing; therefore, they cannot make intentional movements. Newborns movements are either just reflexes or an involuntary response to an external stimulus. So, I guess her pee actions were excusable, and definitely laughable.

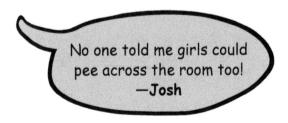

> No one told me girls could pee across the room too!
> —Josh

# TROUBLE WITH NUMBER TWO

Another issue I battled with my newborns was constipation
. . . or so I thought. With my oldest son, he began getting fussy
in a way that we thought was due to constipation. The reason
we went to constipation as opposed to something like hunger
was because his crying usually followed his poop grunts. I can't
explain poop grunts, but I can assure you, you will learn your
child's specific poop grunts rather quickly! So, we bought those
little laxative gels you stick in their rectum, with the hopes of
alleviating his discomfort. My mom ended up being my hero
when she told me his fussiness was most likely from gas, and not
from constipation. She said if I pedaled his feet like he was riding
a bike, it would help stimulate his bowels and he would be able
to pass the gas trapped in his belly We did a combination of the
bicycle pedal and added warm compresses to his belly, and *voilà*!
His crankiness dissolved.

If a baby is constipated and you give them prunes/
prune juice, *leave the diaper on until they have
pooped*. I cannot stress this enough. It only takes
like a max of thirty minutes to work. And trust
me, you do not want to be at the end of a potential
poop cannon.

—Haley

My daughter was born some ten years after the birth of my first
child. Although I had two others between them, when she came
along enough time had passed since I had last given birth that

it felt like being a first-time mother again. People told me that "it's like riding a bike." Well, let me tell you: they were wrong! Although I had picked up some handy tricks along the way, I had also forgotten about many things . . . like baby constipation.

When I thought my daughter was constipated at the ripe old age of one week, I googled home remedies. I learned that if you stick a lubricated rectal thermometer in a baby's rectum, it stimulates the bowels. After a long deliberation with my mom (and attempting the bicycle pedal trick) we tried the thermometer. To my shock, my daughter actually enjoyed the thermometer and let out a funny little coo, but she did poop.

The following day, my daughter had her one-week check up with her pediatrician, and I brought up our poop issues. I told him she had been constipated and what I had done to alleviate it . . . but also told him I was going to need different ideas because I would not be doing that again. The pediatrician asked if she had gone poop after we tried that and asked what the consistency was. I told him it had indeed worked, and it was of normal consistency. He said, "Then she wasn't constipated. She is constipated if she poops out little balls, but if she is solely breast fed, the likelihood of her becoming constipated is very slim." Well thanks for the info doc . . . I wish I would have known this last night!

So now you know! Unless your baby is pooping out balls, he or she is *not* constipated, and there is no need to stick anything up anywhere!

## DOES IT FIT?

My next piece of advice when it comes to changing time falls on the topic of diaper sizes. Figuring out when to move up to the next size is all about trial and error. If it is too small, it leaks. If it is too big, it leaks. Keep a couple sizes handy so you can be sure you have a back-up if it turns out you have the wrong size on baby. For more advice, read down the page to learn my tried-and-true method of figuring out how to know when to move up diaper sizes.

No one told me how a diaper should fit until my son's day care worker pulled me aside at pick up one day and said, "Um, do you think he's ready for a bigger size diaper now?" I was like, "I don't know. What do you think?" She said, "Well, when they start to fit like underwear you typically want to move up a size." I mean, okay, good to know.
—Cindy

By the time my third child came around I had learned that it was time to move up diaper sizes when my baby had a blowout. If the poop is up their back, the diaper is too small. I can tell you that this method works wonders. By the time my fourth child came around, we only had two blowouts total because we had learned to make the quick adjustment to a larger size—as opposed to the two per week we experienced with my first child!

Do not stock up on diapers. You have no idea how long they will be in any one size. Our last baby was in newborn diapers for like a week and a half.
—Ashleigh

My advice here is actually to feel free to stock up on diapers because you can return them. Honestly, I would rather have too many than not enough, because of course you won't realize you are out of diapers until it is one in the morning and the last thing you want to do is make a trip to the store. Fun fact: the barcode will tell you where the package of diapers came from so you can return diapers even if they were gifts.

> An infant can projectile poop across an entire room. Said infant can also projectile vomit across the room. The first time this happened, I laughed so hard I cried.
>
> —Tiffany

## WHAT'S WRONG WITH THEIR POOP?!

Let me start with meconium. Meconium is what a baby poops out shortly after being born. This black tar-like substance is all that stuff they were ingesting when they were still nestled inside your belly. Well, in my experience, they failed to mention that tar-like poop is normal until you're hysterical during your first diaper change. You frantically push the button for the nurses, just for them to giggle and tell you that this is normal for baby's first few days.

> Use a small amount of virgin olive oil on baby's bottom with every diaper change. This prevents the meconium from sticking and prevents over wiping their sensitive little bottom. [It] glides right off. Wish I had known this with my first three children.
>
> —Sarah

If you feed your baby particular items, expect their poop to look a particular way. A baby's digestive tract is much shorter than that of an adult, so they do not have as much time to digest their food. Which means their poop can be the same color as whatever it is they have eaten.

> No one warned me about baby poop after eating bananas. I lived in Africa and thought she had some weird worms.
>
> —Erin

> No one told me that when you feed your toddler mandarin oranges, they come out looking like maggots in his diaper!
>
> —Tara

# GROWING PAINS

Alligator wrestling is a perfect comparison for what it's like to change a toddler. If you read the chapter on gift registry ideas, you read about how hard it is to snap the buttons on the pajamas of a toddler; this is the same concept, except now bodily fluids are involved. I gave up on the changing table as soon as my kids began flipping around, and there were many times where a naked butt waddled out of the room because I couldn't get them to stay still—and baby butts are cute. Occupying your baby's curiosity or attention can help your baby stay still. My go-to method was usually a baby cracker or toy. Really though, I would have given them a Rolex to play with if it would have kept them still long enough to get them changed.

Diaper changing a toddler should be considered a competitive sport. I am convinced that this is the reason people potty train. They just get tired of trying to change the diaper of an upside-down monkey. Do not get me wrong, I love her adorable little butt, but I do not want it in my face as I am trying to put her diaper on.

**—Anonymous**

It is so hard to change a diaper once they are mobile because they flip around like an alligator and waddle their butt away. Adorable but also annoying.

**—Garesh**

# DIAPER RASH

Diaper rash can come from so many things that it is hard to pinpoint what the culprit is, but there are some causes that you can eliminate when trying to find the cause. Teething, high acid foods like pineapple, new foods, new products like diapers or wipes, being in a used diaper for too long, illness, and sensitive skin are all things that will cause your little one to develop those dreaded (and inevitable) diaper rashes. Changing your baby frequently, thick diaper rash creams, and letting your baby roam without a diaper for as long as possible will help clear up rashes.

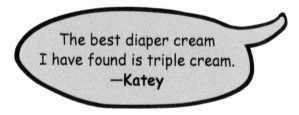

The best diaper cream
I have found is triple cream.
—Katey

As discussed in the gift registry chapter, I am rather partial to butt paste, but at the end of the day you should get what works best for your baby's skin.

# CHAPTER 16

# IT'S SO CUTE! HOW DO YOU PUT IT ON?

Imagine this: You have been kidnapped by terrorists who have forced you to stay awake for days at a time (an actual torture method). Each time you fall asleep, they force you awake with the sound of a baby crying. Your body hurts. You are exhausted. Just when you think you cannot stand it one more second . . . they throw a onesie at you and tell you to put it on a baby who refuses to stay still. That is what it feels like when you own snap or button-up onesies. Maybe there are some moms out there who can handle snaps and bottoms after weeks of sleepless nights, but I am not one of them. In my experience, zippers are the only way.

> Baby clothes are a pain in the butt to put on and take off. Be good to yourself and do not buy the outfits that are cute but take a small army to get on.
>
> —Danielle

> Zip-up outfits are life. Buttons are the devil.
> —Meagan

It does not matter how cute an outfit is. What matters is if you can get that outfit off your child without smearing poop through their hair because they just had a major blowout. What matters is being able to take their pajamas off and put them back on when it is two in the morning, and you have not slept in a month.

> Onesies have the weird shoulders so you can pull them down when there is a blowout instead of over baby's head. Do not ask how many kids I had before I learned this!
>
> —Annie

Yeah, I learned this a couple of kids in. I wish I had known before my first child, as this advice would have saved me the battle of trying to get a poop-laced onesie over my baby's head without getting it in his hair!

> Magnetic onesies are your best friend, especially at three in the morning.
>
> —Lilly

Those outfits that look so darn cute are alright to buy, especially for new moms who still have the energy to take a zillion pictures every day. Just understand that those outfits are meant to be put on right after baby's afternoon nap and diaper change, when baby is in a good mood, and you are not in zombie mode yet. You slap the super adorable outfit on them, take a million pictures, then hurry up and take it off before your child realizes they have something cute on and decides to ruin it. I am quite sure cute clothes cause diarrhea.

Another factor to keep in mind is how quickly babies grow. An outfit that is perfect for them one day may not fit after a week. You may find yourself with several dozen newborn outfits but nothing that fits at six or nine months. Having a baby grow out of clothes they never even wore has always been the worst part of parenting for me.

This was especially true with my daughter. Let's face it: little girls' clothes are so much cuter than little boys' clothes. Before she was old enough to decide what she wanted to wear, I would try to get all her outfits on her at least once before she outgrew them, but it was inevitable that I find an outfit with the tags still on it when I was switching out sizes. Once my daughter was old enough to dress herself or have some say in what she wore, all bets were off. More times than not, clothes moved on to new owners with the tags attached.

> Ain't no one got time to dress their little pumpkin in every cute newborn outfit you will get. Be stern yet kind when people ask what you need. Do not ask for baby clothes. [I] cannot tell you how many brand-new outfits I gave away because she was never able to wear them.
>
> —Christy

> Most babies don't stay in newborn clothes more than a few weeks.
>
> —Jessica

People love to buy baby clothes for the obvious reason: the cute factor. But my advice is to be as specific as possible when people ask you what you'd like when they're trying to buy you baby gifts. Ask for a range of sizes. Ask for zippers, not buttons or snaps. And if you don't need any more clothes, don't be afraid to say so! Any time people asked me, I would tell them the size I was buying at the time, which sometimes meant a size or two higher than she was currently wearing. However, this meant less outgrowing of outfits and less need to make bulk purchases when it was time to move up in sizes.

Nobody told me just how far off birth-weight estimates can be, even by very experienced docs/ midwives. [My] estimates were for an eight-plus pound baby at thirty-six to forty-one weeks. When I delivered after a hard induction, my baby was barely over six pounds at forty-one weeks. I had to go buy preemie clothes after we were released, and those lasted a couple weeks before we even hit the newborn size.

—Julonda

Once your baby hits their toddler years, getting them dressed is like competing in the rodeo. You have to sit on one arm as you try to get the other shoved in a sleeve, all while trying to avoid their feet as they kick wildly. Buy T-shirts and leggings; these are the easiest to put on a bucking bronco.

# CHAPTER 17

# DOES IT EVER STOP CRYING?!

Sometimes babies just cry, and it is not because they do not like you or you are doing something wrong. Sometimes they just cry and there is nothing you can do . . . except maybe cry with them. I talk a lot about my colicky child in this book, presumably because he helped contribute to most of my experiences on the topic of crying, or maybe it is because I don't want other moms to struggle with the issues he and I secretly struggled with because I didn't know how to ask for help.

## EMOTIONAL NEEDS

Think about yourself as an adult for a moment: How many times in your life have you found yourself crying without a reason why? Or there is a reason, but it is so silly you don't want to admit that something so seemingly pointless has brought you to tears? I can think of many times in my life that this has happened to me, and since having Layla, this happens to me more and more often. So how can we not expect this same behavior from our babies? Babies who were, just weeks or months prior, taken from the wet, dark, quiet environment they had known and thrust into this new world. A world in which they can easily be overstimulated, feel lonely, or require an amount of attention that they cannot ask for.

So, let's talk about overstimulation. Overstimulation is when one cannot cope with the level of sensation or external influences they are experiencing, such as noise and touch. For babies, this can happen far more quickly than it does for most adults. Being passed around from person to person, loud or crowded places, and new environments can easily overstimulate your baby, which can lead to one of those crying spells where nothing you do seems to make baby happy. Stimulation is amazing for a baby, but if your baby has been overstimulated, take them somewhere quiet and familiar where they can regain their sense of safety.

Another thing we often don't realize with babies is that they can feel just as lonely as we do—they just don't know how to express that loneliness or know what to do to fix it. You may find that your baby's physical needs have been met and they are not hurting, yet they are still inconsolable. You may find that simply holding your baby or rocking them will calm your baby, but the moment you put them down, they are right back to crying. This is often due to their need for attention or their feelings of loneliness. You cannot over-hold your baby or spoil your baby, so hold them as often or as much as you want.

If your baby's need for attention surpasses yours (which happens to us all at some point in our parenting journey), ask friends or family members to spend time with you and baby. Company will allow you to focus on someone other than your baby and gives your baby someone that cannot wait to hold and cuddle them. Baby wearing is also ideal for these situations. Your baby will always be happiest when they are close to you, but it is not always logical to carry around your baby. Wearing your baby can give your baby the closeness they crave and the freedom you desire.

# PHYSICAL NEEDS

You may think that this section goes without saying: obviously we all know what a baby's physical needs are . . . but do we? Sure—feed them, change them, temperature, find out if they are sleepy . . . right? I wish. But before I go into the physical needs we may not always talk about, let's talk about the ones we already know.

Feedings. Ah yes, make sure they aren't hungry. Check, next one. Right? Wrong! Yes, make sure your baby is fed, but be cognizant of what you are feeding them and how. Are you breast-feeding? What you eat is passed on to your baby, and although you may love extra spicy Thai food with extra jalapenos, your little one won't love the acid reflux it gives them. Bottle-feeding? Bottle-feeding tends to give little ones more air, so make sure you are burping your little one after eating—especially bottle or breastfeeding if they were crying in the moments leading up to said meal.

This next one is my biggest (read that in big, bold emphasis), *biggest* pet peeve. I will be out and about on a Texas summer day, sporting my shorts and tank top, when I see a fellow mom dressed similarly to me. As always, my eyes wander down to the sweet little angel bundled—yes, bundled—in their car seat or stroller. I'm talking a fuzzy blanket, hat, socks, long sleeves, etc. It takes everything I have not to walk up to mom and ask them if they're cold. When they tell me they aren't, then I can proceed to explain to them that their baby isn't either, and in reality, is overheating in that nice little cocoon they've been bundled in for that freezing 102-degree day.

Your pediatrician will *hopefully* tell you this before you ask, but if not, let me break it down for you: dress your baby to the level that you are dressed, unless of course you are weird like me (or my youngest boy), then dress your baby in what is relevant for the temperature. For instance, you wouldn't wear a big fuzzy jacket in 100-degree heat, so don't wrap your baby in a fuzzy blanket. When my youngest son was in elementary school, I would literally get hate mail from his principal because he never had a jacket on in the winter (it was in his backpack), because the little dude just likes cold weather. But you can bet your butt that, as a baby, he had that big fuzzy blanket wrapped around him when it was cold. All that is to say, dress your baby for the environment they are in.

Whew. Now that I got that off my chest, we can move on. One thing that contributes to crying is teething. Sweet, wonderful, horrible . . . teething. Teething is probably the least enjoyable thing about having a new baby. Right when you finally think you have the hang of things and created a schedule that works, your baby starts teething. Suddenly, the baby who was finally sleeping through the night is up screaming every two hours. All the tricks you had picked up along the way suddenly do not work, and your heart breaks into a million pieces every time you hear that cry of pain coming from your sweet angel.

You will notice that most of the recommendations are the same, just with some variation, such as the frozen items or teething tablets. While frozen bananas worked for baby one, maybe it will be a frozen washcloth that works for baby two. If one method does not work, do not lose faith, just try another. I lived by Dr. Talbot's teething tablets, which are tiny little pills that dissolve immediately. There is no concern about choking, and one will provide quick relief.

When I noticed that my baby's gums were swollen and red, I would give them something frozen to chew on, whether it was fruit, a wet towel, or a teething toy meant to be frozen. The cold from the frozen item helps lower inflammation and swelling, which provides relief. Amber necklaces were not around (or maybe not popular?) when my kids were babies, so I do not have firsthand experience with them, but I have many friends that swear by them. Here are some other tips and tricks parents swear by to help your baby get through those terrible teething moments.

- Freeze a wet washcloth and let your baby chew on that.
- Teething straws and tubes are amazing. We started my daughter on them at three months and she loved them, plus as a bonus she gained the best hand-eye coordination.
- Put teething meds on the nipple of the bottle or try flavored pacifiers.
- Amber teething necklaces and bracelets are made from Baltic amber and meant for pain relief. In theory, when the baby's warm body heats up the amber, a small amount of succinic acid is released and absorbed into the baby's bloodstream. The succinic acid is meant to have an analgesic effect.
- Talbot's chamomile tablets or Hyland's oral relief tabs provide quick pain relief.
- Freeze foods they enjoy. We found waffles, bananas, and even celery were successful. Even simple ice can help.
- Copaiba essential oil is also very soothing.
- Freeze breast milk in a plastic pacifier.

# COLIC

Another big struggle for new parents is what to do when *nothing* seems to help. You've checked everything you can. Baby isn't wet, isn't hungry, isn't sick, isn't uncomfortable . . . and *still* won't stop crying. These prolonged spouts of crying for no apparent reason could be an indicator that your child is colicky. Colic is stressful for parents and presumably for the baby, but it is not harmful to your baby, despite their wails sounding like they are in pain. Colic cries are extreme, loud, and inconsolable, often leading parents to feel like there is something wrong with their baby. The good news is that colic is predictable and there are strategies to help your baby. The bad news is that there is nothing that "cures" colic: your baby just grows out of it somewhere around three or four months.

> That colic is real, and it sucks, and everyone still manages to survive it. Whatever it is that soothes the colicky baby, just do it! If you have to stand up and rock her for three hours every night or drive the car around until she falls asleep . . . do it.
> —Michelle

I talk about colic throughout all the chapters in this book because I experienced it so heavily with my youngest son. I hope that if you end up with a colicky baby you can take something from this book, apply it to your baby, and find that it works. I drove my son around every night before bed, we used the dryer method (strap baby into the car seat, put it on the dryer, and turn the dryer on), and even put him in his car seat in a dark closet when he was too over-stimulated from all our attempts to calm him. You have to do what works for your baby, and unfortunately, I cannot tell you what that is. What I can tell you is this: don't go through it alone. Colic is when the term "it takes a village" really comes into play.

> Sometimes nothing works to calm a crying baby. Don't take it personally.
> —Jill

Sometimes a change of scenery can help. And even if it doesn't make baby stop crying, it might make you feel better to be out of the house—or at least feel like you're doing something besides sitting around with a screaming baby.

As you and your baby get to know each other better, you'll begin to understand what they're communicating with different cries. Even in your most frustrated moments, try to remember that since babies don't speak yet, crying is one of the few ways they have of telling us what they're feeling. You'll begin to identify the angry cry, the hungry cry, the sleepy cry, and so on.

> My baby screams like a pterodactyl when she is angry. It is hard for me to listen to, but I know it's just her way of communicating with me.
> —Garesha

> Someone gave me a onesie with advice on it I'd wished I had with the first two: no baby ever died from crying.
> —Roxanne

# CHAPTER 18

# SHH ... BABY IS SLEEPING

I think your body starts preparing you for those sleepless nights with a newborn when you are still pregnant, because it is increasingly hard to sleep during the last few weeks of pregnancy. I think this hit around week thirty-five for me. I went from sleeping peacefully every night to begging all that is good for just two hours of uninterrupted sleep. If I was not getting up to go pee, I was readjusting the body pillows surrounding my expanding belly or trying to flop over like a beached whale.

Sleeping in one position for too long becomes uncomfortable, but turning over is like trying to roll a ship over on land. And whether you drank one ounce of water or one hundred ounces of water throughout the day, you will pee at least ten times during the night, but be prepared for just a little drop or two to come out each time.

Do not worry though: the final trimester lack of sleep is only temporary. Once your baby is born, you will be able to sleep again—*they* just will not let you. Who are *they*, you ask? Well, in the hospital, "they" means the nurses who come in your room every thirty minutes to check your or baby's vitals. "They" at home refers to that sweet little bundle you just spent the last nine months carrying in your womb.

> Enjoy your sleep before they arrive, because after that sleep is a luxury.
>
> —Jordan

As you read this chapter, you will see a trend in the comments along the lines of "sleep when they sleep." New moms may feel like they need to jump right back into cooking and cleaning as soon as they get home from the hospital. Some may battle severe "mom guilt" when they let those things go. The result is an overtired, emotional mom who is battling postpartum hormonal swings *as well as* sleep deprivation. By the time your second child comes around, you realize those chores can wait. Instead of utilizing baby's nap time to clean, you use it to catch up on some much-needed sleep. As a result, you are better equipped to handle your new baby's constant needs and your own postpartum woes.

> The three hours that baby sleeps at night means you get one hour of sleep at best. Nobody tells you how exhausted that lack of sleep will make you.
>
> —Nicole

I cannot tell you exactly how your baby will sleep. If anybody tries to do so, respectfully tell them to shut up. Every child is different, and all of yours will be too. You will quickly learn that what helped your friend or worked for your first child may not help your current newborn. My first child slept from 8:00 p.m. to 8:00 a.m. every day from the day he was born. Sleepless nights? Nope, we did not have them. He was such an amazing baby that I decided to do it again! However, baby number two made up for all the nights baby number one had let me sleep.

My second child was colicky and therefore did not sleep more than ten to fifteen minutes at a time, ever. His incessant crying became so unbearable that my mom, my husband, and I had to take turns caring for him. The ladies in my church would offer suggestions (all of which I tried) or would take him thinking they had the magical touch that would finally get him quiet. Each time they would give him back still wailing, at a loss for advice or words of wisdom.

No one said what "sleeping like a baby" is really like. They were off beat with that phrase!
—Rosie

My daughter was somewhere in the middle of her two brothers. She did not sleep all night, but she also did not cry all night, so I counted that as a win. The most valuable piece of advice I was given during my first pregnancy was to "sleep when they sleep" (especially as a working mom who was just home for a few weeks). Understand that the chores will be there the next day, laundry can wait another hour, and the dishes will not explode if they are not washed right now. If baby is sleeping and you need some sleep, go sleep!

> For the first few days at least, the baby is only going to want to sleep on you, and if you want sleep, you will do it. If she's like my two-year-old, she'll never stop only sleeping on you.
>
> **—Ashley**

You cannot do anything for your child if you are deliriously tired and overwhelmed. The post-pregnancy hormones are going to have you on a crazy enough roller coaster; you do not need to add sleep deprivation. When I was a single mom, I did not have the luxury of having a dad around to take over the parenting in the evenings, so when people offered to come hold baby so I could sleep, clean, shower, or whatever I needed to do, I accepted their offer. There were times that friends sat in a rocking chair next to my bed holding my girl while I took a much-needed catnap or finally took that shower.

There is no way to give one-size-fits-all advice on how to get a new baby to sleep, but I have compiled a list of methods that have helped me and countless other moms.

- Drive your baby around until they fall asleep.
- Strap your baby into their car seat and set them on a turned-on dryer. The heat, sound, and rhythmic movement tends to sooth a cranky baby.
- I slept with my baby lying on my stomach. This is not recommended by experts, but sometimes it was the only way I could get my baby to sleep.
- One of my babies slept in a baby swing next to my bed. The rocking soothed her, and she was right there when it was time to nurse.

- If you aren't nursing, have a setup next to your bed that includes a thermos of warm water and bottles with pre-measured formula powder so that you do not have to get up to make or warm up bottles every two hours.
- Try having baby sleep in a Pack N' Play at the foot of the bed. Sometimes your baby or young child just wants to be near you.
- A routine can be very helpful, especially for an older baby. If every night is the same—bath time, book while nursing, rocking baby until she falls asleep—then baby will get used to the routine and know when it is bedtime.
- A sound machine, one that covers up other background noise, can be a game-changer. There is nothing like finally getting your baby to sleep just to have them woken up by people talking in the hallway.
- I do not recommend getting up constantly to change your babies' diapers. Only change them if they poop or soak through their diaper. I would always put my baby to sleep in a diaper that was a size larger than what they wore during the day (if they wore a one, they slept in a two). That way the diaper would keep them dry for longer, and I would not have to wake them while they were sleeping.
- Swaddling can also help baby feel safe and secure and improve their sleeping habits.

A final word of advice on sleeping: do what is right for *you* and *your* baby, not what is right according to your friend or family member. Take all well-intentioned advice with a grain of salt and do what works for you.

# CHAPTER 19

# JUST FOR DAD

With all the focus on mama and the new baby, I feel like dads often get the short end of the stick. Nobody is giving dad tips or advice on parenting, they don't get a baby shower (although joint showers are becoming more popular in our culture), and nobody stops to see how dad is doing. So, I wanted to be sure to include not just advice *for* dads, but stories and tips from the perspective *of* dads. The first part of this chapter includes two sections written by special dad contributors. After that, you'll find advice for dads from moms and advice for dads from dads.

## MY SON'S FIRST CRY
*Contributed by Jeff*

The first child is like nothing you will ever experience again in life. Many questions popped into my mind, as I am sure they do for many first-time fathers: Will I be a good dad? Will my wife accept the way I parent? Will my new child look at me with love? Of course, I knew the answers to these questions, but they still flowed through my mind.

The pregnancy part was interesting, to say the least. My wife had specific cravings that could not be fulfilled twenty-four hours of the day, but we made the best of it. I knew she was going through things that I could never understand, from the emotional changes, to the exhaustion of carrying a child inside of her, all the way to trying to be a happy wife. It was tiresome for her, so I needed to pick up the slack and be that support team she needed.

When my son came to us that July night, everything we planned up to that point seemed to zip out and disappear. I had no idea what I was doing, even though we planned it. I was more nervous than she was. So nervous, in fact, that I spilled ice chips on her while trying to feed them to her. She laughed, but I was going insane.

"Is it time yet?" I kept asking. It had only been ten minutes.

I was worried the doctor would not make it in time. I feared that something would go wrong during delivery. The anxiety consumed me as I waited and wondered.

As the morning turned into afternoon, and then afternoon to evening, I became more impatient. Not only was I anxious and exhausted, but I also had not eaten since that morning. My mom and wife encouraged me to go get some food, promising I would not miss the birth of my son while hunting for a sandwich. My wife was only dilated to a five, and my mom said we still had hours to go. The nurse did a quick check to ease my mind and give us an approximate timeframe.

I watched the nurse's face go from all business to excitement as she told us my wife had jumped from being five centimeters dilated to nine centimeters. It was time to have a baby! It was time for delivery, but where was the doctor? Nurses were paging our doctor, but could not make contact.

I tried to stay calm as I frantically thought, *My son is coming, and we need our doctor!* My fears were becoming reality, yet when I looked at my wife she was as calm as could be. I do not know how she held everything together. She should have been the one freaking out, not me, right? Finally, the nurse came back and said our doctor was with another patient doing an emergency delivery, so the on-call doctor would be there shortly.

Wait, no! We had spent months with our doctor; we did not know this other person. He did not know what we discussed with our regular ob-gyn, the decisions we had made, or our plans for our baby's delivery. I had to realize that there was not much we could do at that point. My son was coming into this world regardless of who delivered him. It was time to buckle up and get ready.

Everything we learned in child birthing class seemed to go right out the window for me. There was too much excitement for me to even think about counting like we had been taught. After a few pushes I could see my son's head, and then with a little twist and pull I was looking right at him. I did not know what to think. I was mesmerized by the sight of this little baby who had just come out of my wife. As soon as the rapture faded, the thought that I am sure every dad has popped into my head: he looks like an alien.

I smiled from ear to ear with joy and excitement. I was eager to hold him and feel his warm soft skin in my hands. My son was here, and we were parents. Everything I worried about before disappeared, and a whole other set of worries ensued. But in that moment, hearing his first cry, I was in love.

# DADDY'S LITTLE GIRL
*Contributed by Jim*

When my daughter was born, I remember sitting in the hospital for hours before she arrived. My wife was in the hospital bed having some intense contractions. And there I was, sitting next to her in a semi-comfortable chair watching the Country Music Awards. She had not been paying attention to what I was doing when she suddenly had another intense contraction and looked at me for comfort. She said a few colorful words and phrases, and I turned the television off. My focus was now on her.

The type of contractions and their frequency had caught the attention of nurses, and suddenly the room was filled with people making final preparations for the delivery. In one breath, my wife was screaming in pain, begging to push our daughter out, and in the next breath cursing my very existence. She also kept reminding the entire room of my fondness for country music. (I do not think I have watched the Country Music Awards since then.) At some point, I left her side so that nurses could get to her. Her legs were high up in stirrups, she was bent forward, and the doctor was positioning himself for what I like to call "the big catch." I stood there in awe as my wife pushed and pushed while everyone cheered her on.

During all this commotion, I remember looking down and witnessing my wife poop on the floor. Doing what most young men would do, I giggled. After all, this was my first child, and I was only twenty-four. I had no idea that was going to happen, and no one prepared us.

Finally, we heard a loud cry as our daughter came into the world. In that moment, our lives changed forever. After the nursing team cleaned her and did all the other things they do, they brought her over to me, semi-wrapped in a blanket. They wanted *me* to cut the umbilical cord! I was hesitant at first, but finally took the scissors and did as they asked. The umbilical cord was spongy and firm, which made it difficult to cut. I think I was afraid of hurting her. Once I cut the cord, they took her and finished weighing and measuring her. Then mom got to hold her for what seemed like an eternity. All I wanted to do was hold her and never let go.

They finally brought her over to me wrapped up tightly in her blanket, and I held my daughter for the very first time. Most fathers dream of having a son, but not me. I was on cloud nine when she was in my arms. At that moment, I was already wrapped around her perfect little finger. And I know she felt the same way, because to celebrate the occasion, she peed on me! To this day, I still proudly proclaim that I was the first person she ever peed on.

My wife and baby spent a couple of days in the hospital to make sure baby was latching correctly (apparently that is a thing) and eating. While they were still in the hospital, I placed an enormous cardboard stork in our front yard. Written on the stork in Sharpie was my daughter's weight, length, and time of arrival. I was a proud brand-new papa! After we received about a bazillion briefings, we got to come home.

When we left for the hospital, I never realized that we were leaving our old lifestyle forever. We returned home and suddenly had a tiny human that needed to be taken care of. There was no more leaving the house spontaneously. Going grocery shopping, or just getting out of the house, required extensive planning. Did we have enough food? Did we have enough change of clothes?

Did we have enough diapers? These were just a few of the questions we had to ask ourselves, or our outing would prove to be catastrophic.

Fortunately for me, my wife was breastfeeding, and I did not have to get up as often in the beginning. This changed when she went back to work and started pumping milk. I never had a problem with feeding our daughter, changing diapers, or any other random tasks, but for some reason I was afraid to bathe her. I think part of it was not wanting to hurt her. In my eyes, she was a tiny, fragile thing that I did not want to break. In hindsight, I wish I had given her baths. I missed out on so many precious bonding moments.

## ADVICE FOR DADS FROM DADS

If you're a dad and you're reading this, congratulations! Here are some words directly from the mouths of other dads who have been there, done that, and are here to tell you all about it. If you're a mom with a partner and you're reading this alone, get dad over here to participate in this chapter with you.

> Since it was my ex-wife who did the actual work during the birth, I felt like it was my responsibility to get up for all the diaper changes and feedings, unless she wanted to do it. It was my turn. Now my girls and I have strong relationships.
> —Kevin

Before you start worrying about *after* the baby is home, research how to bring a baby into the world. So many partners do not prepare themselves, so they do not know what to expect. Then they are left with war stories instead of the miracle it is supposed to be. Just relax, trust her body, and work as a team. You must be her support system and her biggest advocate. I have heard so many women say that they did not have their husband's support and they felt robbed of the whole experience. Also, post birth, you take baby duty while she sleeps!

—Andy

Ask some friends and family to sign up on "Take Them a Meal." It is an online meal train system to help new parents in those first few weeks. Provide your wife with snacks or a drink while she is breastfeeding. Do not wait for her to ask if you will take baby duty so she can shower; tell her to go take a shower and decompress (she may get offended at first, but then she will thank you). Carry the car seat. Let her say whatever she wants while she is pushing and be her advocate if she needs anything. Cherish every second; they do not stay little long. The things your children do will bring you more joy than you have ever experienced (even [when they're] writing on the wall).

—Carl

Stay present with your kids. Find things that you both enjoy doing, and sometimes even allow them to make the schedule.

—Sean

When your wife is packing her bag for the hospital, pack [yourself] one too. Include a charger and a laptop (or something to do).

—Matthew

The actual birth was not nearly as bad as I mentally prepared for. We had a C-section, and I got more nervous working myself up to it, but everything went so quickly and smoothly. Just remember that you are at a hospital with staff that do this every day. The hospital we went to averages thirty C-sections a month; there were two others there while we were getting ours. Point being, they are professionals and know what is going on. Go with the flow and get excited for your new baby.

—Ryan

If your significant other must have an emergency C-section, they will have to take her back to prep her, and you will be left alone for around twenty minutes. Even though you are feeling terrible and more helpless and scared than ever before, things will be fine. They know what they are doing, and once they come get you, you will have your prize in your arms in under ten minutes. Long story short, you will feel bad, but in the end, it will be so worth it.

—Nick

Get a baby carrier ASAP. My son will not fall asleep unless he is on one of our chests. The baby carrier gives you mobility and makes you look like the world's greatest dad lol. They are rated up to twenty-five pounds.

—Robert

Your baby is not *her* responsibility. When it is your turn to keep your child, you are not "babysitting" or "watching" your child; you are sharing in your part of parental duties. It also is not her sole responsibility to change all the diapers, do all the feeding, be the primary caregiver . . . Remember, this is a team sport, and you are in this together. Share in the sleepless nights, the colicky baby, the fun times, and the not-so-fun times.

—Brent

The best advice I can give a new dad is enjoy every moment. There will be times that it is so tough [and] you just do not know what to do, but try your best to just cherish it all. You won't ever get that time back with them, and it goes by so fast. I say this as a father of older children and a father of a newborn.

—**Ash**

1. Ask your wife, "What can I do for you?" Offer to take baby so mom can do some things on her own, like shower, pee, or get some sleep.
2. Yes, dads can get PPD, too, so be sure to check in on your friends with new kids. Do not be afraid to reach out if you are feeling off after the birth of your baby.
3. The household chores can wait. If they can't, don't ask your wife to do them. Do them for her or hire someone.
4. Make you partner food when you make yourself food.
5. Be gentle on mom. Having a baby kicks your butt emotionally, physically, and mentally.

—**Dan**

# ADVICE FOR DADS FROM MOMS

I'll be the first to admit, I didn't think about how having a child affected a man until my first husband explained the stress he was feeling shortly after we found out we were pregnant. When I was thinking about the baby's sex, cute clothes, and how to decorate the nursery, my husband was thinking about the financial impact of having a child. While it's completely impossible to include everything a dad would want to know, I've done my best to compile a thorough list of "they forgot to mention" moments to give you a good overview.

> Anything you and your partner say between the hours of 7:00 p.m. and 7:00 a.m. does not count. The sleepless newborn nights will be 100 percent easier [if you give] each other a clean slate every morning.
>
> —Olivia

Personally, I think this is generally great advice, even when you don't have a newborn baby at home! Let me give you a little lesson about the brain. The amygdala is the part of your brain that is responsible for your bodies fight or flight reactions, i.e. it controls your stress responses and the reactions that cause you to either scream and run, or turn around and fight. When you lose sleep, your amygdala is on overdrive, causing you to overreact to the simplest of stimuli. So when baby has kept you up all night, what normally doesn't cause a reaction can be the thing that sends you overboard.

Expect her to need your help and be willing to help. Pay attention to how she does things; this will keep stress-related arguments to a minimum. Trust her intuition when it comes to your baby and do not let outside opinions influence how you feed and care for your baby. When my husband saw that nursing was not working for [me and] my baby, he suggested formula and ignored all the hype about "breast is best." We switched, I cried, my son got fed, and now, fifteen years later, you can't tell him from a breast-fed baby. Fed is best. Better than that, a supportive and observant husband is worth his weight in gold.

—Amy

It is normal for dads to get postpartum anxiety and depression, but not many people know about that. I highly recommend hiring a postpartum doula for the first few weeks after the baby is born to help you all get adjusted to your new normal.

—Carolyn

Learn to ask for and receive help from others. Hire someone to clean and accept or set up a meal train (people bringing you food).

—Jennifer

This is great advice for everyone, but there is a reason it is specifically important for dads. Men have been taught for so many generations that they need to be tough, that they cannot ask for help, and that needing help is weak. It isn't weak to know when you cannot do something on your own; quite the opposite, it shows strength. I feel like women have an easier time asking for help because it has always been more socially acceptable, although it should be just as acceptable for a man.

Give yourself and your partner grace. You are going to be so tired and haggard from the huge life adjustment. You are going to pick fights with each other. Acknowledge that you are doing it because of the changes and sleeplessness. Try not to take it personally, and do not look at it as something wrong in your marriage. It is just a phase, and all new parents go through it whether it's their first kid or fifth. Apologize quicker, forgive sooner, and put things around the house on the back burner so you can spend time with your partner when baby is asleep.

—Katie

Help your wife out when she is breastfeeding. Make her some food or bring her a drink. Breastfeeding takes a lot out of you.

—Jenn

Do not be offended if your baby does not go to you right away, or if mom is the only one that can comfort baby. She was all your baby knew for nine months. Help build that attachment by taking part in daily caregiving, reading to or playing with baby, and creating traditions between just you two.

—Jenny

## STRESS RELIEF TIPS FOR NEW DADS, BY DADS

- Take a walk outside
- Exercise
- Play some video games or any game you enjoy, like darts or pool
- Golf
- Have a drink (like a relaxing beer)
- Build something
- Try going for a solo drive or ride your motorcycle
- Listen to or play music
- Try getting down on the ground and playing with your kids—I would play Legos or cars with my son and soon all those things that were stressing me out disappeared
- Sit on the toilet an extra five minutes—this is the only place in the house where nobody will bother you (unless you are mom)
- Sit by the fire
- Spend time with your family
- Anything outdoors: lawn care, hunting, fishing

- Get a dog (but be sure to check with your partner first)
- Sports, watching or playing

(I kept this in here because I am not a man or a dad, so who am I to say what a man should or shouldn't do. However, as a mom with seven kids, three dogs, and a slew of barn animals, I can say that adding a dog to the mix of a newborn in the house could be a bit overwhelming. Unless maybe it is an older dog? Either way, I wouldn't really jump on the bandwagon of adding more responsibility on top of a baby.)

# CHAPTER 20

# RAISING 'EM SOLO

I always dreamed of having kids . . . twelve of them, to be exact. I would meet the man of my dreams, get married, and proceed to have twelve beautiful daughters. Okay, maybe some of them would be sons. My kids would grow up in a loving family with a stay-at-home mom, homemade snacks, and no fast food. My husband and I would be so in love, and my kids would grow up knowing what it was like to live in a two-parent home, unlike me. I never knew my dad.

Well, it kind of started out the way I had imagined it in my head, the marriage part anyway. I got married young and proceeded to immediately start trying for kids. After a year and a half of being married, we welcomed our first son, followed twenty-two months later by his brother. The first pregnancy was out of the pure, unadulterated desire for a child; the second was a desperate attempt to save my rapidly failing marriage. By the time my second son's first birthday came around, my husband and I had split up.

The first five years of raising two kids on my own and fighting tooth and nail with my ex-husband were brutal. My ex and I could not agree on anything in the courtroom and verbally attacked each other outside of it. If I was not in court fighting for my sons, I was getting visits from Child Protective Services for some unfounded accusation or working extra jobs to make ends meet. It was not what I had imagined, and I spent those years missing out on precious moments with my kids because I was too busy ensuring my ex-husband was miserable.

The only thing either of us did right during those first years was spend holidays together. Whether it was a birthday party or Christmas, we would attend it together so our children did not have to go back and forth, and neither parent missed out. Yet what we did wrong would have lasting effects on our children. We have both spent the following ten years encouraging recently divorced parents to play nice regarding their children, because the children are the ones who stand to suffer the most.

> All you can do is choose to make the right decision next time, and every time after that. Sometimes you will make the wrong one, and you must come back from that . . . but you always come back. Life is a journey, and nobody said it would be easy. Life is filled with so many ups and downs. Those down times make the up times that much better, and soon the ups will start outshining the bad. We all win some and lose some, but in the end, it is all worth it.
>
> **—Amber**

Those terrible years of fighting over our kids made me never want to have another child. I dated throughout the years follow-ing my divorce, but every time the guy began mentioning family and kids, I ran. I did not want to repeat what I had been through with another child. When I got pregnant eight years after my divorce, it came as quite a shock to me. However, there was one great thing about this pregnancy: I was not with her dad, and he had no interest in being in her life.

I thought not having a man involved would make everything easier. In some ways it definitely did, but in other ways it was much harder not having a significant other to share in certain moments, such as ultrasounds, feeling the baby kick, or those days when you just want to cry. Those moments would have been easier with someone else there. On the other hand, things like choosing a name, room décor, a birthing plan, etc., were much easier without someone else around. My daughter's dad told me he could not be a part of her life, and I was fine with that. Having the baby on my own meant that I wouldn't have to go through the fight I did with my boys' dad; she would always just be mine.

I would have friends go with me to ultrasounds and decided my oldest son would be in the birthing room with me and cut the umbilical cord, a tradition usually saved for the dad or significant other. If I got lonely at night, I'd text an old flame to chat with, or snuggle up with my other kids and watch a movie. The only difficulties I faced were my ever-changing emotions and trying to keep those in check while being the only disciplinarian to my two rambunctious sons.

You can scream, cry, holler, get mad, whatever . . . then pick yourself and keep handling your business. Read positive affirmations, drink a glass of wine, take care of yourself. You must know you will be alright; you have to be.

—Anonymous

The reality that I was doing this alone and that I would never have her daddy to share in every moment did not fully sink in until I went into labor. Suddenly I realized it was just me, and there was nobody else to take care of my other kids, hold my hand through contractions, or cuddle our new baby while I got some much-needed rest. Fortunately for me though, people I barely even knew banded together and helped pull me through.

Suddenly there were people there to help that I never even would have thought to ask. The elders' wives at the church would stay with my boys and take them to school. There was someone from church, my work, or my son's football team there to hold my hand and rub my back, and there was always someone around willing to hold my girl while I got some sleep or took a shower. Sure, it was not how I had planned it, but life never is. I learned very quickly that you cannot plan for every moment, and you cannot dwell on what could have been.

> Take life one day at a time. Work on getting your feet under you and into a position where you can provide for you and your baby on your own. Stay focused on loving your babies and the fact that nothing is permanent.
>
> —Shak

As a single parent, I learned to lean on other people and build up a tribe around me. You must take things as they come and live each moment for what it is. Sometimes life was pretty okay, and I could just take things day by day. Other times I had to take life minute-by-minute because my emotions were too hard to control, especially when I was dealing with postpartum depression. Eventually, we fell into a routine and life as a single mom became a wee bit easier.

Sit down and write out a short-term plan [and] a long-term plan. Post them up on your mirror. Each day, focus on taking one step closer to your goals. Remind yourself that every day will be better than the last. Be your own coach.

—Drea

Now, twelve years after my divorce, my ex-husband and I have a great friendship and can co-parent on good terms. I approached parenting my daughter differently because I was afraid to repeat what happened with him, but it turns out my concern was unnecessary. Two years after my daughter was born, her dad and I got married. Now, two years later, we have a beautiful blended family, with a sweet little girl tying it all together.

Had it not been for my years as a single mom, I do not think my relationship with my husband would be as strong as it is. I know without a shadow of a doubt that my relationship with my birth children would not be nearly as incredible as it is now had it not been for the years when we battled our difficulties together, just us against the world. If you are a single parent wondering how you are going to survive, do yourself a favor and give yourself a break. Do not compare yourself to other parents, and especially not to two-parent households. Understand that your situation is unique and being a single parent is the hardest thing any person can go through.

> Get out of the house whenever you can. Fresh air does wonders for the mind.
>
> —Taryn

> Practice primal screaming . . . seriously. Don't knock it 'til you try it.
>
> —Alex

Your life will not look the same as it would if there had been a mom and a dad. You may experience bouts of guilt when you must miss certain moments or events because you are the sole breadwinner in your house. You may have nights when you cry yourself to sleep (yes, even you, men) or stand in the doorway of your child's room crying over what could have been. Allow the tears to come, allow yourself to feel, then stand up, wipe the tears away and tell yourself that there is nobody in the world stronger than a single parent.

> Remember that one day you will look back and say with pride that you did it on your own, that you are the reason your children are the wonderful adults they became. Know that your happiness is worth more than anything in this world because our children need a parent who is happy.
>
> —Kayla

# CHAPTER 21

# BONUS PARENTS

Being a stepparent is . . . stressful. Difficult. Frustrating. Overwhelming. Fun. Exciting. Amazing. We all know the age-old adage "being a parent is the hardest job you will ever have." I would say this is wrong. Being a parent is the *second* hardest job, second only to being a stepparent.

I could write an entire book on being a bonus parent (another term for stepparent), but because this book is for new parents, I will stick to just one chapter. I wish I could say that I have conquered the challenge of a blended family, and that by reading this chapter you, too, will suddenly know the secret. But alas, when it comes to blending a family, I think the story is never over and the work will always be ongoing. But I've learned a few lessons from my own experience and I'm here to share what advice I have. I do think stepparents and stepchildren alike will giggle at the stories I am about to tell, because they, too, have "been there, done that."

When my second husband and I first met, he was—*le sigh*—perfect. Like seriously, he opened his mouth, and it was like the sun broke through the clouds. Imagine a cartoon with the birds flying around and singing, and the girl gets big hearts in her eyes . . . yeah, that was me. Then I found out he had four kids. Four.

Not one. Not two. *Four* little humans that I *knew* would drive us apart. How did I know this? Well, he wasn't the first single dad I had ever dated, and those relationships all ended the same way, with a big fat "Thanks, but no thanks!" How these other dads parented was just too different to how I parented. This fact always led me to bail.

But I met my second husband later in life (I say "later," although I am only thirty-two, I got an early start with kids) and by the time we met I had quite a bit of life experience. At the time, his kids were ten, seven, and the twins were three years old. My two boys were nine and seven. And yes, I must admit it, I judged a man with kids despite having two of my own. We dated for two years before introducing my sons into the relationship, and for three years before introducing his kids. All the while, I secretly worried our happily-ever-after would end the moment I met his kids.

Now, five years and one beautiful baby later, our family of nine has blended into a cohesive mix. I must be kidding, right? How could the person so hesitant to meet someone else's kids have a blended marriage that is actually working? I will explain! This cohesive mix of yours/mine/ours came together after many tears, some counseling, and a *lot* of com-promises. And by compromises, I mean we both had to grow the hell up.

The advice in this chapter comes from my own experience as a woman currently living the day-to-day battles of a blended family. I also sought advice from other parents who either have a blended family currently or raised a blended family whose kids are now all out of the house. Most importantly though, this advice comes following my and my husband's decision to go to counseling. Counseling taught us both how to love more deeply, forgive more quickly, and self-reflect more thoughtfully (both of us were used to judging others but never ourselves). We learned that those mountains we were once willing to die on were actually just molehills . . . and weren't worth the strain on our relationship.

My husband and I made the decision to get pre-marital counseling because this was a first marriage for neither of us, and we wanted to give this new marriage the best chance at being successful. We decided we would take the year before our marriage to attend counseling and work through a couples' book that had been recommended to us. However, as it often does, life interfered with our plans. Due to some unforeseen circumstances, we moved our wedding up. Suddenly, we were both thrust into a new life with all these kids and two completely different styles of parenting.

My parenting style mirrored that of a drill sergeant building new recruits up to be soldiers. This included daily chores, helping with dinner, eating what was served, severely restricted screen times, keeping a clean house, and a *lot* of yelling whenever I got home from work and the kids hadn't followed through with my perfectly laid out rules. Brent's parenting style, on the other hand, was far laxer. His kids had no chores and no limit on screen time. He made special meals for his picky eater and cleaned the house himself. There was also far less yelling in his household. These two parenting styles did not mesh well, and the nine-person household was chaotic to say the least.

In the very beginning, remember you are not the parent or disciplinarian; you are this new entity that your significant other has decided to team up with, and the kids didn't have a say in it. Slowly ease into things, and be on the same page with your significant other when it comes to things like discipline and dividing up chores. If you do not agree with something your significant other is doing, be a united front in front of the kids. Discuss why you don't agree once the kids are out of earshot. If you have a high-conflict biological parent situation, be patient, thick-skinned, and don't ever let their child hear you say anything negative about their parent, despite what their parent has said about you. Most important: love one another, have each other's backs, and love those kids despite how difficult things can be sometimes.

—Amanda

About a week into our marriage, we decided to attend the counseling appointment that we had made before deciding to move up our wedding. Although the appointment was for "pre-marital" counseling, I think we were both desperate to try anything that could help us. Our problems were already mounting. His daughter thought I would starve her when I said, "you get what you get and you don't throw a fit," at dinner time (a method I had employed with my own kids for the last ten years). We had a needless yelling and bag-packing argument about house décor. Two weeks into our marriage and one week before I would have signed the divorce papers (just kidding . . . mostly), we headed off to marriage counseling.

Our counselor was a mouse of a lady who couldn't say her Rs and told us she hadn't raised her voice in forty years. I spent the first hour of our session (yes, it was multiple hours) convincing myself that I didn't like her and secretly making fun of the way she said "Bwent," instead of "Brent." But then something incredible happened: she started telling Brent that he was wrong in the way he saw some things at home and began making suggestions about how he could improve. I left that first counseling session feeling vindicated and excited for our next session, expecting our counselor would once again tell my husband that I was the superior parent. But our next appointment unfolded very differently. Instead of telling Brent how he was wrong, she turned to me and pointed out where I was in the wrong. It went this was for the six months; some days she laid into Brent, other days it was me.

Some sessions we would start out holding hands and by the end were sitting as far as we could from one another. Yet little by little, we stopped sweating the small stuff. Soon my husband and I began to be a united front to our children instead of two people allowing their kids to get between them. By the end of the sixth month of counseling, we had learned so much and had grown both as a couple and as parents. I would highly recommend early marriage counseling for any newly married couple or any new parents, but even more strongly urge blended families to see a counselor. Counseling offers a third-party point of view that can keep molehills from turning into mountains.

Counseling is what took us from being "stepparents" and "stepchildren" to being "bonus parents" and "bonus children." Our counselor taught us how to compromise without giving away a part of ourselves. She taught us how to love one another in a way we hadn't loved each other before. She taught us to give each other grace. Most importantly, she walked us through how to be bonus parents to our stepchildren. One of the main things we both had to learn was that what had worked for us individually before may not necessarily work now.

Clearly define each other's role in the family, and clearly communicate that to the children.

Listen to your children's comments, take a moment to understand how they feel, and see if there is anything you need to change. We are not perfect, and we are all learning as we go. Know that everything is subject to change.

—Heather

We had to learn to compromise and pick our battles. Shockingly enough, the hardest place for us to do that was with food. Brent's kids had been allowed to be picky and only eat certain things. For one daughter, that meant only macaroni and cheese or spaghetti noodles. At every meal, his ex-wife would cook their picky eater her own food. In my home, my children were not allowed to be picky eaters; they had to eat whatever they were served. If they didn't eat it, they didn't get anything else.

When Brent and I got married, we immediately saw the chasm between his way and my way in regard to food. In the beginning I was completely unwilling to budge, and this stubbornness hurt not only my relationship with the kids, but my relationship with my husband as well. I began to have anxiety whenever his kids were due to come over. Meanwhile, Brent's daughter thought if she didn't eat whatever I made that I would make her starve. My unwillingness to compromise was taking a toll on our family and my marriage.

Through counseling and communication, we were able to come to an agreement that not only worked for Brent and me, but also for our children. We even included our kids in the discussion because they needed to understand why we were struggling with such a seemingly minute issue. It was important for us that our daughter understood that she was going to have to begin expanding what she was willing to eat because she wasn't the only one affected. It wasn't fair for her to have her own special meal while the other kids had to eat something they didn't necessarily love. There was also no way on the planet that I was going to make everyone their own food every night. Some days we were lucky when one of us had time to cook anything at all.

> Make sure the children involved know that you and your partner are a team. This will help tremendously when following through with rules, discipline, routine, etc. Depending on age, you could make them a part of that process.
> —Michael

We ended up making a decision that worked for our whole family. When we cook, we make meals that include something all the kids like. They may not like everything in the meal, but there is at least *something* they will like. For instance, when we do "taco night," it consists of making beans and meat, setting out tortillas and all the fixings for burritos, and then letting the kids assemble what they want. The younger girls will all make quesadillas, our two picky eaters usually eat a bean burrito, and the rest of us make tacos. I no longer felt like I was compromising my values, and the kids don't feel unheard. Mealtime is no longer a subject of contention, but an enjoyable time together.

We have also seen growth in the daughter who was the pickiest eater. About a year into our marriage, I asked her to start trying one bite of everything we made, and soon we began to see her like more and more foods. My son also enjoys our style of compromise because he is no longer forced to eat foods he doesn't like. Instead, he's able to choose foods that suit him more. In the end, we all win because we've learned from one another and have all become more flexible.

> This cannot happen in all situations, but try to have a good co-parenting relationship with your spouse's ex. We do a family dinner with my husband, his ex-wife, her new fiancé, my stepdaughter, and myself a couple times a year. This makes our daughter feel more comfortable having a relationship with all of us and doesn't feel like she is in the middle of some war. We try to plan activities and holidays together when we can. This really makes my daughter feel special.
>
> **—Shanna**

Being a bonus parent has taught me to relax and enjoy life more than I ever have before. Don't let what you have previously decided is good parenting stop you from actually *being* a good parent. I was a single mom for so long that I spent more time preparing my kids for adulthood than I did enjoying their childhood. Compromising for my bonus children didn't only help my relationship with them, it also helped me with my own kids. They became more relaxed around me, and I around them. So yes, being a stepparent can be stressful, difficult, frustrating, and overwhelming . . . but it can also be fun, exciting, and amazing.

Just keep in mind that these tips and advice are what worked for me and the other bonus parents I talked to; that does not mean that every piece of advice will work for you. Some blended families do better with clearly defined boundaries, whereas other families work better when the lines are a bit more blurred. For my family, we do best when we both take on full parenting roles. This means one parent will do the disciplining whether it is their biological child or their stepchild. It also means listening and lending a hand when the other parent is feeling overwhelmed, used, unheard, etc.

As always, take these tips and mold them into something that works for you and your unique tribe.

# CAVEAT TO THE FOLLOWING TWO CHAPTERS

People are hardwired with their own personalities and attributes. There are some qualities and traits that we tend to attribute to boys and some that we attribute to girls. However, it's important to remember that every individual is unique and will have their own combination of traits and a unique way of expressing themselves. Plus, there are those individuals who don't fall into traditional gender roles, as well as those we lovingly refer to as LGBTQ+. I would have written a chapter about children who identify this way or about same-sex parents/spouses, but I recognize that I simply do not have enough experience to accurately speak on behalf of the LGBTQ+ community. As you read these chapters, please understand that I write about "boy traits" and "girl traits" under the assumption that these babies were born within more typical gender norms simply because that's been the experience I have to draw on.

# CHAPTER 22

# BOYS! JUST LIKE GIRLS, BUT HARDER TO KEEP ALIVE

I write this chapter under the assumption that the mom of a new boy is reading this while sipping on her fifth cup of coffee, hiding in the bathroom, and secretly wondering if there is something wrong with her adorable, sweet, fun-loving, rambunctious, destructive, and very loud son. One moment he is the sweetest little cuddle bug you have ever met . . . and the next he is trying to convince you that he is a sociopath. I hope by the time you are done reading this chapter, you are laughing and thinking about all the special (grey-hair-inducing) moments only a little boy can give you.

My first child was a boy. Let me preface this by saying that I had never planned on a son. As a young woman, I babysat little girls in our church, dreamed of the day I would have my own daughters, and kept a running list of what I would name them. I didn't keep a list of boy names because I didn't think I needed any boy names; my plan was to have girls. So imagine my surprise when the ultrasound tech told me that my soon-to-appear little bundle of joy was a boy. I knew nothing about little boys and hadn't planned on needing to learn.

Now, let me follow up by saying that my first son not only taught me all about little boys, but also became the reason I prayed for more sons. He was born on a Tuesday night after an induction and three hours of pushing. He came out a fat little cherub weighing a solid eight pounds, one ounce, and could have easily passed for a one-month-old. When the doctor held up my newborn son for all of us to see, Kenny lifted his head off the doctor's hand and looked straight at my husband and me. That moment right there should have told us that we were on the ride of our lives with this one.

Kenny did not follow the norms of a "typical" baby boy. Baby boys tend to wake up more frequently throughout the night and, when compared to girls, wake up far fussier. But not Kenny. He slept from eight in the evening until eight in the morning from the day he was born (granted, he was latched on to one of my boobs for most of this time as well). He never cried; if he soiled or wet his diaper, whatever, he just kept trucking along. He was the happiest baby you could ever meet, and he never met a stranger.

I enjoyed that baby boy so much, I decided to have another one (though really, this second pregnancy was also an attempt to save my failing marriage). Shoot, if all boys were this easy, I would have fifty! This time, when it was time to learn the gender, I prayed for a little boy, and was ecstatic when the tech told us that my prayers had come true! My pregnancy with my second son was as uneventful as the first, minus a second rogue sack breaking during my second trimester and scaring everyone. However, once this baby was born, he was as different from his brother as two children can be.

My second son, Andy, was everything you don't want to experience in parenthood (I wrote more about this in the chapter on bonding). He was nothing like what I had expected a little boy to be based on my first son. I worried there was something wrong with Andy from the moment he came out of my womb;

not only did he hate everyone (including me), but he also cried for the first six months of his life. My husband and I were so focused on our colicky new baby that we missed that fact that our older son, Kenny, was becoming a toddler . . . and toddlers, my friends, are what separates the weak from the strong.

The first thing that Kenny began to do as a toddler that drove me insane (although my husband swore was perfectly normal) was sleep with his hand in his diaper. I nearly vomited the first time I took my toddler's diaper off in the morning and he had an erection, which even his pediatrician swore was perfectly normal. His obsession with his male genitalia did not go away until he was out of those toddler years (or maybe he just hides it now). Now when my friends have little boys, I get to share a private chuckle with a new mom when she confides in me that her toddler son woke up with an erection or won't keep his hands out of his diaper.

> Be prepared to be peed on all the time for the first couple of months. When they get older, be prepared to find pee all over the bathroom once they start going on their own.
>
> —Jamie

But that's not all. Kenny was the only child I knew (remember, I only had experience with girls up until his birth) who could fall off a fence, scrape his knee, or break a bone, and just laugh about it. I even took him to our doctor after his third emergency trip to the hospital, because I was truly afraid there was something mentally wrong with Kenny (don't judge me, I was very young).

The doctor tried to be sympathetic and understanding, but I couldn't help but notice his poorly veiled attempt to hide his laughter as he listened to my plight.

The pediatrician explained to me that although my son did not *appear* to feel physical pain, he most certainly did feel pain—and more importantly, he felt emotional pain. The pediatrician explained that males tend to have a higher pain tolerance and a tendency to be more reckless. He said that male and female brains are hardwired differently, and a male brain is hardwired to be more active (I have since learned that this isn't necessarily true, but at the time it made me feel so much better).

What's most important is that I learned not to compare my son to the girls I had babysat as a kid, and began to enjoy learning about little boys. Oh, and I also put poison control on speed dial. However, my rambunctious little toddler wasn't done teaching me about boys yet. As soon as he was old enough to move his arms, he broke everything in sight. Toys? Broken. Household goods? Broken. The irreplaceable whatever-it-was that I refused to put away because "my son would learn not to touch it?" Yep. Broken.

I couldn't understand how I could buy a toy and it could be broken by the time we got to the car. Why did he just have to break *everything*? I would work myself up and get so angry. As a stay-at-home mom, I felt like he was wasting the hard-earned money that had been spent on that toy. You could tell when he went from rolling to crawling to walking, because the broken items in my house came from higher and higher up. After a while, it didn't matter how high we put things. He could climb like nobody's business.

Nowadays I look back at those moments when I was too busy fretting over "spilled milk" to enjoy his toddler years. I can no longer recall what items he broke, though at the time they were so near and dear to my heart. The lesson I learned is that things are replaceable, but people and moments are not. Kenny is the reason I was able to cherish every moment with my daughter as a toddler. One day I blinked, and my little terror was a grown man. And guess what? He grew out of his destructive phase.

> Be prepared for drama. Just because they are boys does not mean there is no drama. Be prepared for sneaky attacks that they call "hugs" or "cuddles" that turn into wrestling matches. Also, be prepared to be hit by flying toys and nerf bullets, or step on broken toys or Legos. Don't be surprised when you have Lightening McQueen driving up and down your head and body while you are trying to eat. Get ready for sweet hugs, sloppy kisses, smelly farts, and random animal noises.
>
> —Evana

Now let me just say, my Google searches for the phrase "is my son a sociopath" didn't really start until the day my ex-husband let me sleep in when he went to work. I woke up later than usual, in a panic because Kenny wasn't in bed (we co-slept). I ran out of my room and heard him giggling on the other side of the house, followed by a giant crash. What I saw when I entered the kitchen mortified me at the time, but now makes me crack a big ole smile. My rascal of a son was sitting on the oven in his diaper. In his hand, he clutched a knife from the knife block, and he had all the teapots I had been collecting lying on the floor. I watched in horror as my son threw said knife at the teapots, breaking another one. He giggled, I bawled . . . it was a good time. Now this story is one of my (and his) favorite ones to tell.

Another one of my favorite boy mom memories is the time I decided to get a side job selling Avon to help with the expenses, since we were a single income home. I was sitting on the floor going through my orders, separating the makeup based on who had bought it. I got up to use the bathroom and, in the little amount of time I was gone, my son opened *all* the packages of new makeup and proceeded to use the contents to draw all over both himself and his baby brother. By now I had gotten the hang of my little hellion, and this time stopped to snap a picture of his handywork before cleaning up his mess. To us, that picture is now worth more than the two hundred (or more) dollars of makeup he ruined.

My second son was the complete opposite of his brother. He was opposite of every boy stereotype I had ever been told about . . . and continues to be. Andy was the epitome of the perfect toddler. Maybe he was making up for those first six months of crying. That little boy didn't even go through a "terrible twos" phase. He was quiet, delicate, and serious. If he ever broke a toy, it was a complete accident, and not something to be repeated. He reacted far more to physical pain than his brother, but showed no emotion when it came to emotional pain.

As my two boys got older and began understanding things better, we learned they reacted very differently to different kinds of punishment. The oldest would bawl his eyes out if you told him that you were disappointed in him, but would laugh if you spanked him. The younger brother would tell you to get over it if you told him that you were disappointed in him, but would bawl if you even tapped his rump. Those two crazy boys are now fourteen and twelve, and still as different as night and day as they were as babies. They are also still the most incredible thing to ever happen to me.

As many minor heart attacks as my oldest son gave me, and as many tears I shed as I tried to learn what was "normal" for boys, and as much frustration I experienced when they were little, none of this compares to the love I received from my little boys. Nobody cuddles better than a little boy, nobody loves on their mama like a little boy, and nothing makes you feel more loved or beautiful than when your son tells you he loves you or that you are beautiful. Even now that my sons tower over me and are double my weight, their cuddles melt my heart.

> Boys are always hungry. The older they get, the worse it gets. Pretty soon your shopping cart will look like you are preparing for a king's feast.
> —Cassandra

The bond a parent feels with their son is something that cannot be replicated. As parents, I really believe we love our male and female children different, at least I do. I feel a fierce bond with all my kids, regardless of their sex. With my sons, I feel a heart-tugging love when I see them growing up. I want to push them out of the nest and watch them spread their wings. With my daughters, I feel a territorial love for them. I want to protect them and tuck them under my wing and never let go.

I didn't realize how much my boys had taught me until I got married and welcomed Caleb, my new oldest son, into my life. I had the opportunity to teach his family something they didn't know about boys. Caleb is so vocal and outspoken when he feels anger or feels slighted, whereas our girls get quiet and cry. I laughed when he told us his mom says he has anger issues, and that my mother-in-law said he was prone to anger. I enjoyed educating them on how a boy's response to things can be vastly different to a girl's response.

All this to say, boys may be a little more destructive than girls or find more joy in breaking things than swaddling them, but there isn't something wrong with them. I ended up putting my oldest son in sports; his high pain tolerance and fearlessness actually made him a naturally talented athlete. Your son does not have anger issues because he chooses to vocalize his feelings or raises his voice when he is feeling overwhelming emotions. Don't make your son feel like there is something wrong with him for how he communicates, instead just encourage him to continue communicating in ever-healthier ways.

Our sons are all teenagers now. Whether they were the perfect baby or hell as a baby, the perfect toddler or Houdini the toddler, they all grow up to become men. In some ways they are so much alike, even the non-biological brothers. They have all hit the same stages as preteens and teens and have had the same struggles (one day I will write a self-help book for parents of twelve-year-olds). Yet they are so astronomically different at the same time.

The best thing we can do for our sons is not compare them to other people's kids, to girls, or even to their own siblings. We must love and respect our children for their differences and the traits that make each of them unique. Cherish every single one of those big, dirty, too-rough, overwhelming hugs that your little baby boy gives you, because one day he won't fit in your lap anymore. Don't criticize a boy (or man) who shows emotions, and don't try to mold their communication methods into how you think they should be. I understand that communication goes both ways and that the relationship between the communicator and listener is twofold, which means communicating in a way that both parties can feel comfortable talking and listening.

The best way I can explain this is if I give you some background on my husband's oldest son, Caleb. When Caleb communicates, he raises his voice, he gets passionate and animated, and often-times *sounds* like he is angry at the person he is communicating. However, as the listeners, we have learned to understand his passion while speaking for what it is, and not take it personally. Yes, he could learn to communicate better, or I could accept his way of communication and not expect him to change to better suit my listening methods as a woman. The advice I will leave you with is this: do what is best for your child, whatever is going to benefit them the most in future relationships, school, work settings, and communication.

# CHAPTER 23

# GIRLS! DELICATE LIKE . . . A BOMB

My daughter has been night-and-day different than my sons since the moment I conceived her. My husband would tell you that I cried when she was conceived, but I don't remember that. I am not typically someone who would be so emotional as to cry after sex! I'd like to say that was the one and only time I got emotional over something small, but that instance was just the first of three years of random emotional outbursts. Not only did my daughter cause me to become more emotional than I had ever been before, but she also helped my body to begin producing estrogen again. Because those "female" emotions were newer to me and I never had any sisters, raising a little girl has been a unique challenge.

> If you have a boy already, just know your love and bond with your daughter will be much different than the love and bond with your son. One hundred percent equal, but different. Invest in something to hold your bows. Dress them in all the girly, ruffled things you want because dressing them doesn't last for long. Oh, and prepare to be broke. Girl things are so much cuter than boys' stuff!
> —Caitlyn

Carrying a baby girl inside your body makes your estrogen levels go haywire in a way that carrying a little boy does not.[1] On top of all the extra emotions that estrogen created, I also had morning sickness from day one with her. I can't say I carried her any higher or lower than my boys. I was always told you carry boys up front and high and girls down low and kind of allover, but this wasn't my experience. I also felt so different in my body. I felt . . . beautiful. My skin was soft, my hair was thick and full of life, my nails grew faster than ever, and I just felt good. That is, until she was born. All those amazing pregnant-with-a-girl bonuses left the moment she was born, leaving me with just the extra emotions to contend with.

> My girls slept through the night early and reached their milestones a bit earlier compared to my son. They were also calmer and a way more balanced than our son and wanted to do things on their own, whereas our son needed more support or help. Girls play (things like animals, dolls, and painting) for hours. Their attention span isn't nearly as short as a baby boy's. They see little details and differences. As well, they feel how moody their mommy is. When I feel sick or sad, they know it always and they take care.
>
> —Ester

As a baby, Layla wasn't particularly different than any other baby. She slept well, waking up often to eat, and nursed like a champ. However, I wish someone had given me a heads up about newborn baby girls and how they differ from little boys.

When my sons were born, we were taught how to pull the penis foreskin back to clean them. However, I wasn't given any insight into the norms of a little girl. One of those that shocked me is that newborn girls can have a minor "menstrual cycle," a false menses caused because of the drop in estrogen after birth. This bleeding is mild, pinkish, and only lasts around ten days . . . but I sure wish someone would have mentioned it.

The second thing I wasn't warned about was the swelling newborn girls experience in their labia after birth. This swelling goes away within two to four weeks, but not before a new mom freaks out and rushes her baby to the pediatrician! But once we got the physical scares out of the way, it was smooth sailing until she got a little bit older and way feistier. I am so glad I had a husband who was experienced with girls; he had already gone through the toddler years with three other girls.

I had three boys, then a girl. She was a lot quicker to reach all of her milestones and was probably my easiest baby, despite being two months early. Not sure if that's a girl thing or not! I know their language is usually more advanced than boys.
—Angie

I had to ask my husband "Why is she doing that?" at least once a day for about two years as I got to know little girls. Either she was crying over nothing or giving me sass I didn't even know could come from a one-year-old. My husband would just laugh and say, "That's what girls do." One day Layla was playing upstairs and got hurt, so my husband went to check on her and brought her down to me to cuddle. I did what I have done for my kids for the past two years: I checked that there was no bleeding, patted her on the head, and sent her on her way.

Layla just stood there with her little bottom lip quivering, looking at me like I had killed her puppy. My husband, in his infinite wisdom, came back over and said, "Babe, she isn't a little boy. You can't just pat her on the head and send her on her way. You need to cuddle her." He brought Layla back over, placed her in my lap, and wrapped my arms around her. She and I sat there with my arms wrapped around her for a few minutes until she decided she was better. Then she jumped up and ran back off to play.

> My significant other swears our daughter is bipolar, but I know it is just a girl thing. She can go from laughing one minute to crying the next, then back to laughing! I'm a first-time mom, but I've been around babies all my life, even special needs babies. It's really just learn as you go.
>
> Girls have such wonderful personalities! My daughter has definitely taught me patience. She truly is my joy!
>
> —Nicole

I still don't react when Layla falls or gets minor bumps and scrapes. Most of the time I joke with her when she gets hurt, saying something like, "You can't open the door with your head!" However, my husband has taught me to recognize it when my little girl needs a little extra love. I have also learned to help our older girls to not get so emotional about everything. My girls are so much more sensitive to physical and emotional pain, harsh tones, and tough situations.

Outside of being far more sensitive than my boys, Layla is also incredibly independent, dramatic, and over-the-top in everything she does. She reminds me on a daily basis that she is a "big gul," then falls asleep tucked into my arms like the baby she is. She is also a daddy's girl and has everyone in the family wrapped around her sweet little finger. She knows how to get her way! Now it is with a playful little giggle when you are trying to be mad, though as a baby it was by making herself so angry she would vomit.

The best advice I can give any new mom of a girl is to be patient. Your girl will push your boundaries, assert her dominance, and drive you insane. However, if you let her, she will teach you love, patience, and a deep gentleness. The love you feel for her will be unlike anything you have ever experienced in your life. You will love her until it hurts. Not more than you love your sons, but a different love nonetheless.

# A FINAL NOTE TO THE READER

I hope you enjoyed my book and were able to laugh at my blunders and take some great notes. Although I have been a medical professional for the bulk of my adulthood, this book is not intended to provide medical advice or replace your doctor; the medical information is merely placed in my book to help new moms have a slight understanding of some of the things happening in their bodies. The intentions of this book are to encourage new parents and help them see the light at the end of the tunnel, as well as making light of some of the moments in parenting that are bound to happen, but are not exactly delightful in the moment. Try to remember: as you are going through your journey of pregnancy, birth, and childhood, that this moment is just a blip in your very long story, so try to enjoy each moment . . . and when you cannot enjoy it, laugh at it. When all else fails and you cannot laugh, grab some tissues (and probably a pad) and have a good cry. Parenting isn't easy, but at the end of the day, it is the most incredible adventure, and you get to be on it.

# WORKS CITED

**Chapter 11: Bonding**

1. Center for Women's Health. (2021). How low estrogen can affect your body. https://www.cwhwichita.com/blog/how-low-estrogen-can-affect-your-body

2. Chisholm, Andrea. (2020). The role of estrogen in your body. *Verywell Health*.https://www.verywellhealth.com/what-is-estrogen-and-what-does-it-do-to-my-body-4142677

3. Shroff, Anita. (Reviewed by). (2020). Forming a bond with your baby—why it isn't always immediate. *WebMD*. https://www.webmd.com/parenting/baby/forming-a-bond-with-your-baby-why-it-isnt-always-immediate#1

4. Halliday, Josh. (2016). One third of new mothers struggle to bond with their baby, research shows. *The Guardian*. https://www.theguardian.com/lifeandstyle/2016/jun/06/one-third-of-new-mothers-struggle-to-bond-with-their-baby-research-shows

**Chapter 12: The Joy of Breasts**

1. Boi, B., Koh, S., & Gail, D. (2012). The effectiveness of cabbage leaf application (treatment) on pain and hardness in beast engorgement and its effect on the duration of breastfeeding. *National Library of Medicine*. https://pubmed.ncbi.nlm.nih.gov/27820535/

## Chapter 14: Sexy Time

1. Moltsen, Mads. (2017). Marriage reduces testosterone in men. *ScienceNordic*. https://sciencenordic. com/denmark-mens-health-videnskabdk/ marriage-reduces-testosterone-in-men/1445183

## Chapter 25: Girls! Delicate like . . . a Bomb

1. Graham, Sarah. (2002). Differences between boys and girls evident three weeks after conception. *Scientific American*. https://www.scientificamerican.com/article/ differences-between-boys/

# BIBLIOGRAPHY

Ayers, S., & Parfitt, Y. (2014). Transition to parenthood and mental health in first-time parents. *Wiley Online Library.* https://onlinelibrary.wiley.com/doi/full/10.1002/imhj.21443

Boi, B., Koh, S., & Gail, D. (2012). The effectiveness of cabbage leaf application (treatment) on pain and hardness in beast engorgement and its effect on the duration of breastfeeding. *National Library of Medicine.* https://pubmed.ncbi.nlm.nih.gov/27820535/

Center for Women's Health. (2021). How low estrogen can affect your body. https://www.cwhwichita.com/blog/how-low-estrogen-can-affect-your-body

Chisholm, Andrea. (2020). The role of estrogen in your body. *Verywell Health.* https://www.verywellhealth.com/what-is-estrogen-and-what-does-it-do-to-my-body-4142677

Graham, Sarah. (2002). Differences between boys and girls evident three weeks after conception. *Scientific American.* https://www.scientificamerican.com/article/differences-between-boys/

Halliday, Josh. (2016). One third of new mothers struggle to bond with their baby, research shows. *The Guardian.* https://www.theguardian.com/lifeandstyle/2016/jun/06/one-third-of-new-mothers-struggle-to-bond-with-their-baby-research-shows

Jenkins, Roberta. (2017). Testosterone levels decrease in men who get married, increase in men who get divorced. *PsyPost.* https://www.psypost.org/2017/08/testosterone-levels-decrease-men-get-married-increase-men-get-divorced-49437

Moltsen, Mads. (2017). Marriage reduces testosterone in men. *ScienceNordic.* https://sciencenordic.com/denmark-mens-health-videnskabdk/marriage-reduces-testosterone-in-men/1445183

Shroff, Anita. (Reviewed by). (2020). Forming a bond with your baby—why it isn't always immediate. *WebMD.* https://www.webmd.com/parenting/baby/forming-a-bond-with-your-baby-why-it-isnt-always-immediate#1

# ABOUT THE AUTHOR

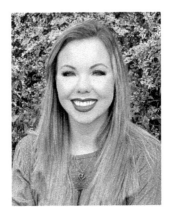

Tiffany Parker is a mother of seven kids ranging from teenagers to toddlers. Tiffany has nearly a decade of experience as a first responder and emergency manager, and has earned a dual master's degree in emergency management and homeland security, as well as a bachelor's degree in public administration and emergency management. Her role as a mother and bonus parent has taught her valuable experiences that she now uses to help other parents going through the same scenarios. Tiffany's degrees, decade of experience as a first responder, and role as a parent allow her the opportunity to pave a path for future generations by sharing her experience through humor and candidness. Tiffany currently focuses her efforts on motivational speaking, writing, and education.